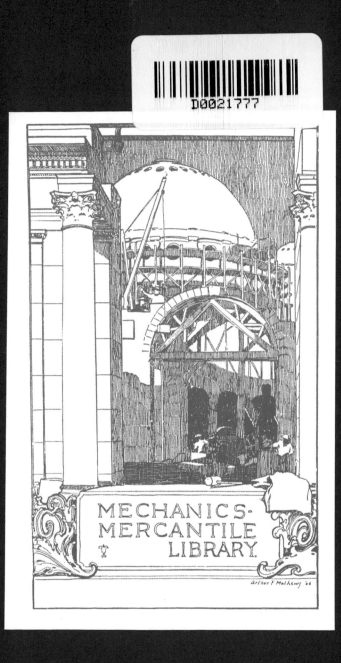

MECHANICS-
MERCANTILE
LIBRARY.

Arthur F. Mathews '06

Good Housekeeping

The Supermarket Diet

Good Housekeeping

The Supermarket Diet

JANIS JIBRIN, M.S., R.D.

Hearst Books
A Division of Sterling Publishing Co., Inc.
NEW YORK

Good Housekeeping

Ellen Levine	Editor in Chief
Susan Westmoreland	Food Director
Delia Hammock, M.S., R.D.	Nutrition Director
Richard Eisenberg	Special Projects Director

Library of Congress Cataloging-in-Publication Data
Jibrin, Janis.
   The good housekeeping supermarket diet : your shopping list for delicious & healthy weight loss / Janis Jibrin.
      p. cm.
   ISBN 1-58816-468-3
      1. Reducing diets—Recipes. I. Title: Supermarket diet. II. Title.

RM222.2.J524 2005
613.2'5—dc22   2005046385

10 9 8 7 6 5 4 3 2 1

Published by Hearst Books
A Division of Sterling Publishing Co., Inc.
387 Park Avenue South, New York, NY 10016

Good Housekeeping is a registered trademark of Hearst Communications, Inc.

www.goodhousekeeping.com

For information about custom editions, special sales, premium and corporate purchases, please contact Sterling Special Sales Department at 800-805-5489 or specialsales@sterlingpub.com.

Distributed in Canada by Sterling Publishing
c/o Canadian Manda Group, 165 Dufferin Street
Toronto, Ontario, Canada M6K 3H6

Distributed in Australia by Capricorn Link (Australia) Pty. Ltd.
P.O. Box 704, Windsor, NSW 2756 Australia

Printed in USA

ISBN-13: 978-1-58816-468-1

ISBN-10: 1-58816-468-3

Contents

Foreword

Whether your goal is to drop some pounds or just maintain your weight, I want to wish you the best of luck. Buying *The Supermarket Diet* from *Good Housekeeping* is a great start. Unlike fad diet books, this one doesn't require complicated mathematical calculations. You don't have to eliminate entire food groups or concoct complicated recipes. And you won't need to shell out extra dollars just to eat right. In fact, our meal plans feature convenient, healthy foods you can easily find by pushing your shopping cart down the grocery aisles. The delicious recipes come straight out of the *Good Housekeeping* kitchens, so you know they're tasty. The exercise recommendations are simple, and I promise you won't need to set aside hours at a time to follow them. In short, this is a diet book for people like you and me.

I've heard *Good Housekeeping* readers complain that the diets they've tried left them hungry. Some gave up because the food choices were limited and boring. And other diets haven't worked because it took too long to see results. You won't have any of those problems with *The Supermarket Diet.*

If you stick to our program, you'll enjoy the recipes, feel full after meals, and will probably lose up to 3 pounds a week at first, then up to 2 pounds a week after that. To help you along the way, we've included the "15 Secrets of People Who've Lost Weight Successfully." Their tips will make it even easier to reach your goals.

Don't forget to check out our website (www.goodhousekeeping.com) for additional useful advice about dieting and fitness. Its message boards let you talk about your experience on *The Supermarket Diet* and pick up tips from the book's author, Janis Jibrin, as well as from other dieters.

Happy eating!
Ellen Levine
Editor in Chief
Good Housekeeping

Part One
Cruising Down the Aisles toward Weight Loss

1 Shop, Eat, and Lose: How *The Supermarket Diet* Works

When's the last time you had a home-cooked meal? If it's been awhile, maybe that explains why you're not happy with the number on the scale. If you do cook and are still overweight, then it's time for a cooking makeover. Either way—home cook or (soon-to-be-former) take-out fan—you're going to whittle down your waistline with *Good Housekeeping*'s slimming, satisfying meals. Plus you'll be in and out of the kitchen quickly; most meals in this book take just 10 to 25 minutes to prepare and call for ingredients you may already know and love. Finally, you have in your hands a guidebook not only to weight loss— there are zillions of those—but also to a slimming way of eating that you can keep up for life.

Make your own food, and you've got the power—the power to slim down. Eat out or take out, and they've got the power—the power to make you fat! Cooking your own food—the right food—is key to slimming down and staying that way. It doesn't take scientific research to tell you that restaurant and take-out food can hit you with lots more calories, unhealthy fats, and sodium than meals made at home can. For instance, the Texan Chicken Burger with a side of beans (page 109) has just a fraction of the calories, saturated fat, and sodium of a fast-food burger and fries.

"But I don't have time to cook!" you say. That's what my clients say, at first. OK, you don't have time to cook elaborate lunches and dinners, but, c'mon, you've got 10 to 25 minutes, the average time it takes to prepare *The Supermarket Diet* recipes. It takes that long to find a parking spot, wait for your takeout, and drive home.

"I don't know how to cook!" (another favorite of my clients). If you're serious about losing weight, you need to develop a few cooking skills. And trust me, preparing any one of these recipes is easier than many other chores you'll do that day.

How about this one? "I can't afford fancy ingredients, and I'm not into running around to specialty stores for trendy foods." You've got a point, and you've come to the right place. *The Supermarket Diet* is all about *convenience:* easy-to-find foods that are right on your local supermarket shelves and easy-to-prepare recipes. If you're a gourmet, you too will find plenty of recipes to love.

And, finally, "I can't take another fad diet." Hallelujah! You should never be duped by a crazy fad diet again. *The Supermarket Diet* is just the opposite of faddish. This plan lets you eat *normal* food. Cereal or toaster waffles are among the breakfast choices. Tuna fish salad sandwiches or Cuban-Style Black Bean Soup (page 67) are typical lunches. Pizza or pork medallions with mashed potatoes count among dinner choices. The meals are balanced and packed with nutrients, so you're not only losing weight but also helping protect yourself against heart disease, cancer, diabetes, and other chronic diseases. You'll also feel energized because of the plan's satisfying balance of carbohydrate, protein and fat. And, yes, you get to have chocolate, peanut butter, and beer!

Because this *isn't* a fad diet, it's not promising "30 pounds in 30 days!" or "Lose belly fat first!" or all the other promises you've heard elsewhere. But if you stick closely to the plan offered in this book, you'll probably lose ½ to 3 pounds a week at first, then a weekly ½ to 2 pounds after that. Generally, the more you weigh, the more you'll lose. Heavier people lose more weight at the beginning than lighter people, sometimes up to 5 pounds in one week. Some of that weight could be water weight. And no matter what your weight, you'll probably drop more pounds the first few weeks, then settle into a slow and steady loss in the weeks and months to come as long as you keep up your healthy eating and exercise habits. I'm also convinced, that once you get in the swing of this plan, you'll feel that weight loss is *doable,* that it's *manageable.*

That's because the food tastes good, it's familiar, and the recommended exercise is not overly demanding (taking walks and doing a little muscle building). Remember, I'm a dietitian working with *Good Housekeeping,* so you know the advice is sensible and effective!

WHY YOU ARE OVERWEIGHT

The reasons you're too heavy may be a little different than why your friend and that guy in your office are overweight. As scientists start uncovering the genes that contribute to obesity, it's increasingly clear that there are many genes involved, and that diet and exercise habits play a big role. Some scientists believe there are four levels of susceptibility toward becoming overweight or obese.

1. A single gene has gone awry, virtually guaranteeing obesity, but this is very rare.

2. You could have a strong genetic predisposition that programs your slow metabolism or gives you faulty signals so you don't know when you're full. However, this doesn't guarantee that you'll become overweight; you can outsmart the genes with proper eating and exercise habits. But you've got to be more vigilant than most people.

3. You have a slight genetic predisposition. You can get away with more food and less exercise than the person with the strong genetic disposition, but you've still got to watch it.

4. You're genetically resistant. Genetically resistant people who don't eat sensibly can gain some excess weight, but they won't become obese.

You probably fall into category 2 or 3. *This is not an obesity death sentence,* but it does mean that you'll have to take your food and exercise habits very seriously, developing a plan you can stick to for life. That's the beauty of *The Supermarket Diet:* It's so flexible and normal that it works with your lifestyle.

WHAT'S OVERWEIGHT?

The mirror is a pretty good indicator of whether you're overweight. But is your weight putting you in medical danger? The more body fat you have, the higher your risk for heart disease, diabetes, and some types of cancer. Scientists have come up with a formula that is a fairly reliable measure of body fat. The formula is called the Body Mass Index (BMI). Use the BMI chart in appendix 1 on page 260 to pinpoint your current BMI, and find out what a healthy weight is for you. (Don't worry, according to the BMI, a healthy weight isn't model thin!)

The BMI is a formula that takes into account weight and height and fairly accurately estimates whether you're carrying around too much body fat. It falters in two extreme cases: People who are heavy because they're very muscular (like pro athletes)—but not fat—might have a BMI in the overweight zone. And people who look normal weight but are so out of condition that they have a high percentage of body fat and low percentage of muscle might be light enough to fall in the healthy weight zone. But for the vast majority of people, the BMI is on target. As indicated on the chart, a BMI of 24.9 or below is considered a healthy weight; 25 to 29.9 is overweight, and 30 and above is obese.

Another way of determining whether you're carrying around an unhealthy amount of fat is by taking a tape measure to your waist. A waist measurement greater than 35 inches for women, or more than 40 inches for men is linked to a higher risk of heart disease and other chronic conditions.

If you are overweight, use the BMI chart to help set your weight goal. Make it reasonable: How about, for starters, dropping down one BMI number? For instance, if you're 5 feet, 5 inches and weigh 168, that's a 28 on the BMI chart. Going down to a BMI of 27 would mean losing 6 pounds. That reasonable goal won't put you under so much pressure that you give up under the strain. Then you can work your way down to the next BMI number. Keep in mind that a relatively small weight loss—10 percent of your current weight—will help lower your risk of developing diseases associated with obesity. This is true for both men and women.

HOW *THE SUPERMARKET DIET* WORKS

With this diet you get three different plans. You can do them in sequential order or jump right into the plan that seems best for you. Each plan offers moderate carbs, moderate fat (about 30 percent of calories), and moderate protein.

1. A two-week 1,200-calorie-per-day Boot Camp, with daily meal plans. This low-calorie level will help you lose weight more quickly than the other levels. However, it might be too low for you, especially for men, and you may feel too hungry. If the Boot Camp continues to feel uncomfortably low in calories after three or four days, skip it, and jump right to Keep On Losin'. Men should skip Boot Camp and start the diet with Keep On Losin'.

2. Keep On Losin' is a 1,500-calorie-a-day plan you can follow for months, even a year. It's *very* flexible. Instead of menu plans, you get to choose any breakfast, lunch, dinner, and snack from long lists. No chance of getting bored with the same old foods. This should be a satisfying calorie level that will help you shed ½ to 2 pounds a week. However, if it's still too low, you can try the Stay Slim Maintenance plan, or alternate between the two.

3. Once you've lost the weight, or if you want to take a break and maintain your weight before losing more, the Stay Slim Maintenance plan is your ticket. It's 1,800 calories a day, low enough to prevent weight regain. If you're a man, especially an active man, you will continue to lose weight on the Stay Slim plan; to maintain weight, increase your caloric intake to 2,100 calories a day. Women may even continue to lose weight on the Stay Slim plan, but slowly. This is also a great plan if you are already at a good weight and need discipline to help stay that way.

Feeling deprived is no fun, and it's what makes people give up on diets. Sure, a little deprivation is part of any successful endeavor: You wouldn't have a flush bank account if you bought everything you wanted, just as you wouldn't have a svelte waistline if you ate everything you wanted. But big-time deprivation is the death knell of many weight-loss efforts. In response to hunger, or monotonous meals, or long lists of forbidden foods, many dieters turn around and binge their way back to their old weight.

So, better to lose weight a little more slowly on a satisfying number of calories than be miserable on too few calories. This means you can choose any of the three calorie options. You do *not* have to start with Boot Camp if experience tells you that consuming only 1,200 calories a day makes you crazy. But if you're really feeling good on 1,200 calories, then go for it! Ditto with the 1,500-calorie Keep On Losin' plan. If you start with the 1,800-calorie Stay Slim plan, you'll still lose weight if you diligently follow the exercise program. It might be slow weight loss, but this isn't a race. (Remember the alternative: If you weren't losing, you might still be gaining weight.)

No matter which plan you're on, exercise is part of the deal. Weight-loss books and programs that proclaim "Lose weight without exercise!" are a bunch of baloney. Studies of "successful losers," those who have lost weight and kept it off, find that these people are physically active. *The Supermarket Diet* offers a doable, gentle-yet-effective walking program, along with pointers on other ways to burn fat. Remember, in order to lose a pound of fat in one week, you need to burn 500 calories more each day than you've been doing. It's much easier to do this by cutting 250 calories from your meals and burning 250 calories through walking or another activity than by dieting alone.

GOOD-BYE LOW CARBS!

You've probably figured out by now that this is *not* a low-carb diet. Now that a slew of research studies have shown that low-carb diets work no better than balanced approaches, there's no reason to recommend them. And there are plenty of reasons not to recommend them:

- Research shows that people often drop out of low-carb diets. For instance, in one year-long study, low-carb dieters lost more weight in the first few months than those on a moderate-carb diet. However, on average, the low-carb group stopped losing weight around the six-month mark while the low-fat/higher-carb group continued dropping pounds for the rest of the year. I see many of these "low-carb refugees" in my office. After losing weight, they get bored with the whole thing, go back to their old eating patterns and, sadly, often wind up heavier than when they started.
- Low-carb diets frequently skimp on fiber, vitamins, minerals, and other healthful compounds found in grains.
- It's not low-carb but *good-carb* that works. Proponents of low-carb diets say that they lower insulin levels and prevent the blood sugar swings that trigger appetite and increase body fat. Well, guess what? Eating high-fiber "good" carbs such as oatmeal, beans, vegetables,

whole-wheat pasta, and the like does precisely the same thing. In fact, studies are starting to point to "low-glycemic-index" diets, those that include "good" carbs, as perhaps the best way to lose weight and maintain weight loss.

HELLO BALANCE!

The Supermarket Diet allows bread, dairy, meats, a few sweets—basically *all* foods—in moderation. It is a very balanced approach, both in terms of getting lots of vitamins, minerals, and other nutrients and in the way you'll feel when you leave the table. The fruits, vegetables, and dairy (or soy milk) offer plenty of nutrients (although I recommend a multi-vitamin/mineral tablet for complete coverage). To make meals as satisfying as possible, they all contain protein, carbohydrates, and fat. Protein is a natural appetite suppressor; carbohydrates (especially the "good" carbs in *The Supermarket Diet* meal) keep your energy up hours after eating; and fat slows stomach emptying, keeping you fuller longer than fat-free meals do.

So, the reason *The Supermarket Diet* works is that you're eating balanced, satisfying meals at calorie levels that promote weight loss. Many fad diets boast that you can eat as much as you want, that calories don't matter. More baloney! A careful examination of these diets shows that people wind up eating about 1,500 calories a day; that's why they lose weight! There's no way around it: To drop pounds, you have to drop calories.

BECOME A SAVVY SHOPPER

You'll emerge from this program not only thinner but also a lot more nutrition-savvy. That's because the book shows you how to understand food labels and find healthy foods at the grocery store (and how to leave the fattening foods behind). Then, at home, you'll have a kitchen stocked with staples that can quickly be turned into a healthy meal.

A WINNING ATTITUDE

Weight loss, if you've ever attempted it before, can be challenging. But like most challenges, it can be incredibly rewarding. The secret to success is attitude. With the right mind-set and dedication to the plan, you can develop a healthy lifestyle.

So begin this program right now, before buying even one item of food, by making a decision. Your decision is to make weight loss a priority. Then give yourself the time to shop wisely at the supermarket, prepare meals (they're easy, I promise!), and get some exercise. Making nutrition and exercise a priority—clearing the space in your life—is critical for success. It may mean asking another member of your family to do a few more chores so you can take walks, or getting up earlier in the morning so that you can fit in some exercise before you start the rest of your day. It will be worth it, and you know it!

Good luck, and enjoy every bite!

2 The Svelte Kitchen

It's 6:30, you're home from work, or you've just had a long day shuttling the kids around, you're hungry, and the last thing you feel like doing is starting a meal from scratch. You open the freezer, no frozen dinners left. You open the fridge: wilted lettuce, questionable-looking cheese, a cluster of condiments. So, you pick up the phone and order a pizza. That's OK once in awhile, but you're never going to lose weight—much less feel energized and healthy—on nightly dinners of pizza, fast food, or other quickie takeouts.

Now let's reshoot the scene with a kitchen that's even minimally stocked. You check the fridge, and there's a bag of prewashed spinach leaves and some eggs. In the freezer you've kept a loaf of whole-wheat bread. (Bread in the freezer? Yup, it stays fresher and better-tasting that way, especially if you don't consume it quickly.) In the pantry, there's some olive oil. Five minutes later, you've got a spinach omelet flanked by two slices of whole-wheat toast and just one pan to clean. Voilà! A 400-calorie, nutritionally balanced meal under your belt. Or, instead of eggs, maybe you found a can of garbanzo beans and some curry powder. In just about 5 minutes, your whole-wheat toast is soaking up a delicious garbanzo-spinach curry. (And if you have them, onions or garlic would make this even better.)

A large part of eating healthy is having the right foods in your kitchen. (The rest is all about overcoming emotional eating, as outlined in chapter 8). If you don't have the time or inclination to cook, the "right" foods might be healthy frozen dinners, eggs, prewashed greens, canned tuna, fruit, whole-grain cereal for breakfast, and a few other staples. While you can lose weight on restaurant food, it's a lot trickier. Unless you order grilled chicken or salmon, steamed vegetables, salad with a little dressing on the side—and how boring is that day after day?—you're probably ordering too many calories. Studies show you wind up with more fat (especially artery-clogging saturated fat), sodium, and calories when you eat out than when you cook at home.

So, seize back calorie control by making your own meals. Your first step: a kitchen stocked with slimming basics. This chapter will tell you exactly what should go into your cupboards and what to throw out. With these standbys, you can whip up a healthy meal in no time. (You'll find more shopping lists for the Boot Camp and Keep On Losin' menus in chapters 3 and 5.) But if you always have these items handy, you'll never be able to use that "There's nothing healthy to eat" excuse again!

Foods to Have on Hand

If you have an empty fridge and bare cupboards: Fill 'em up! And if your kitchen and pantry are overloaded, chuck your scale saboteurs and replace them with the items on this list. (To help you part with the troublesome foods, see "Throw 'Em Out!" on page 32.)

ICE QUEENS: BEST FREEZER STAPLES
Frozen Dinners
Thanks in large part to Mexican, Asian, and Indian dishes, frozen meals have come a long way from the institutional-tasting TV dinners of your childhood. Check frozen entrée labels for 300 to 400 calories and go for at least two of the following:

- Saturated fat: 5 g or less
- Sodium: 600 mg or less
- Fiber: 5 g or more
- Protein: 14 g or more
- Carbs: not much more than 45 g

Boot Campers, you need about 400–450 calories total for each lunch and dinner. On the Keep On Losin' program it's 400 calories for lunch, 500 for dinner. It seems like you'd lose weight quicker on skimpy 270-calorie diet frozen dinners, but that strategy backfires. You'll get too hungry, setting you up for overeating later. So, if the frozen meals are lower in calories than recommended, then bolster with other foods.

Here's what a nutritionally balanced meal looks like: at least 1 cup of vegetables; ½ to 1 cup of pasta, rice, or other grain; and about ¾ cup beans or 3 ounces animal protein. If your favorite frozen meal doesn't cover all these bases, shore it up yourself. For instance, if you love the low-fat chicken-broccoli Alfredo, but there's not all that much broccoli, just steam fresh broccoli or microwave frozen broccoli on the side. Or perhaps you like a great mushroom barley pilaf that happens to be short on protein. Before serving, simply toss the pilaf with ½ cup chopped tofu or cooked chicken.

Best Frozen Vegetables
Keep on hand a bag of frozen broccoli or broccoli/cauliflower/carrot or other broccoli-based mixes. Use them in stir-fries, pasta, and as side dishes. Another great pick: edamame, which are young, green soybeans. Steam the whole pods and sprinkle with coarse salt before serving (don't eat the shells). Or, use the lightly steamed, shelled beans in stir-fries, salads, or rice dishes, or serve them marinated. They're high in protein: ½ cup covers half of the recommended 25 daily grams of soy protein to help lower cholesterol. Frozen spinach is also a nutritious choice and can be substituted for fresh spinach in a pinch.

Best Breads
Buy bread or tortillas with whole wheat as the first ingredient and at least 2 g of fiber per slice or per 75-calorie tortilla (about 5 g fiber for a 120-calorie tortilla). Bread keeps best in the freezer. Take out just as much as you need and heat in the toaster oven. A good rule of thumb: Keep your total bread/tortilla/bagel intake to under 190 calories per meal. Read labels carefully because some of these baked goods are enormous, and the calories apply to just half a slice or even a quarter of a bagel.

Fast-Frozen Meat and Fish
Veggie Burgers. Check labels for at least 12 g of protein per burger; these are the ones with soy as the first or second ingredient.

Chicken. Skinless boneless chicken breast or lean ground chicken burgers will save you time after time. Before freezing breasts, wrap each one separately in plastic wrap so you can defrost them as needed. Avoid coated chicken breasts; the extra calories aren't worth it. Keep raw breasts, patties, and precooked chicken in the refrigerator for when time is really tight. (See pages 205-207 for nutrition details.)

Fish. Since frozen fish can taste and smell fishier than fresh, experiment with different types. Salmon is a nutrition star, loaded with omega-3 fats and linked to heart health, mental health, and a healthy pregnancy as well as alleviation of rheumatoid arthritis symptoms. Frozen wild salmon burgers—available in health food stores and some supermarkets—are low in contaminants that may plague farm-raised salmon sold in the fresh fish department.

If you prefer white fish, go for the unbreaded fillets, which are lower in calories and trans fat than the breaded fillets and fish sticks. However, most of these products use pollack, a low-fat fish with very few omega-3s.

Best Frozen Fruit

Always have a bag of frozen blueberries, which rank among the most antioxidant-rich fruit. (For details, see page 87.) Blackberries, raspberries, and strawberries also contain antioxidants and are loaded with fiber. Frozen mangos and frozen cantaloupe are very tasty and a great source of the antioxidant beta carotene. Buy frozen fruit unsweetened and add your own sugar or honey if necessary. Frozen fruit is perfect in yogurt-based blender shakes.

REFRIGERATOR BASICS

Dairy Musts

Choose fat-free or 1% milk, saving you up to 70 calories per cup over 2% or whole; calcium-enriched soy milk is another excellent choice. Forgot milk? Keep around an emergency carton of aseptically packaged soy or regular milk. Stock lowfat plain yogurt to top baked potatoes, blend in smoothies, cut with mayo, or have as a healthy snack with fruit and nuts. Parmesan lasts for months, especially if it's not grated. Or, grate a hunk and store half in the freezer where it lasts for months. Reduced-fat (not fat-free, ugh!) Swiss and Cheddar are loaded with calcium; buy 'em sliced or grated.

Attention Shoppers! ➤ Berries

Fresh or frozen unsweetened berries score high in nutrition. Here's how to pick the best ones:

Blackberries and raspberries: Get the plump, deeply colored berries with no sign of mold.

Blueberries: They should have a little give, somewhere between hard pellets and slightly soft. Too soft means overripe or aged. Avoid wrinkly or moldy berries!

Strawberries: Choose plump, firm, deep-colored strawberries with bright green caps and no signs of mold or soft spots. Ripe strawberries have a distinct strawberry fragrance, but the scent might be muted if cold.

Store berries in a breathable container (plastic or paper basket, not in a plastic bag) and cover the container loosely if you don't plan on eating them within 24 hours. Raspberries are particularly fragile; don't wash them until just before using or the water that clings to the berries might make them slimy.

Fresh berries freeze beautifully with the following technique. Wash and dry them well on a double paper towel–lined cookie sheet. When berries are dry, keep them on the cookie sheet and freeze for 4 to 5 hours. Then roll them gently into resealable plastic bags and return to the freezer. They don't clump, so it's easy to reach in and take out just the amount you need.

Vegetables

All vegetables are good for you, and the more you eat, the less room you have for high-calorie foods.

Long-lasting staples. If you're not a frequent shopper, stock up on the longest-lasting fresh vegetables: carrots, celery, onions, radishes, and root vegetables. They'll stay perky up to two weeks as long as you keep them covered. Sun-dried tomatoes keep well and make a great addition to salads, pizzas, dips, and many other dishes. Save calories by buying them plain, not marinated in oil. Some brands are softer and more tender than others. The harder, drier type is easily revived by soaking in a little water.

Greens. Collards, kale, mustard greens, spinach, and Swiss chard aren't as long-lasting as the produce mentioned above, but they're nutritional musts. As for salad greens, buy what you like. To get out of a greens rut, if you haven't tried arugula and watercress, give them a whirl. The same compounds that make them so good for you also give them their distinctive peppery bite. In a mixed salad, "blander" vegetables such as avocados, sweet peppers, and tomatoes help balance the tangy taste of arugula and watercress.

Greens thrive in cool weather, even taste a little sweeter. Since there are fewer bugs in winter fields, these greens produce fewer of the bitter compounds that act as natural insecticides. Southerners should be able to find greens at the farmer's market all winter long; try interesting varieties and the tender, less pungent "baby" greens. They are simple to prepare: just wash, cut off the tough bottom stems, and with water droplets clinging, place in hot olive oil seasoned with garlic, ginger, hot peppers, or other spices.

Squash and root vegetables. Picked in the fall, these vegetables are fresher in the cooler seasons than in the spring and summer. Acorn, butternut, and other orange-fleshed squash are high in the antioxidants carotenes. Feeling adventurous? Try horseradish, rutabagas, and turnips for a change. These are cruciferous vegetables, with the accompanying beneficial plant compounds (phytonutrients) (see the "Crazy for

Attention Shoppers! ➤ Buy Your Greens

Leafy green vegetables are so loaded with nutrients that the National Cancer Institute recommends eating them daily. Nutrient credentials include lutein and zeaxanthin, which help protect the eyes from cataracts and macular degeneration, the leading cause of blindness. Spinach is loaded with lutein as are many of the cruciferous green vegetables.

Cruciferous" box above). Beets get their color from compounds called betalains, antioxidants that protect oxidation of LDL, or bad cholesterol (oxidation is one of the steps to artery clogging). Sweet potatoes supply four to six times the daily requirement of vitamin A. Potatoes with skin are a good source of fiber.

Fresh Fruit

Infrequent shoppers take note: Grapefruit, lemons, and oranges last for weeks, offering cancer- and heart disease–fighting vitamin C and citrus bioflavonoids. Grate lemon and orange rinds into fruit salads and rice dishes and into the batter for home-baked bran muffins, and you will soak up limonene, a proven cancer fighter. Apples and pears, especially fresh ones from farmer's markets, should stay firm and tasty for two weeks in the fridge. Fruits with less longevity but bursting with antioxidants: berries of any kind, cantaloupe, kiwis, mangoes, and papaya.

Superior Spreads

Use reduced-fat mayo (about 5 g fat per tablespoon) in tuna or chicken salad and trans fat–free margarines to spread on toast.

Eggs

A fast and easy way to bring protein into your meal. *The Supermarket Diet* uses large eggs.

Jarred Minced Garlic

An instant heart-healthy flavor infuser for stir-fries, sautés, salad dressings, and marinades. (Or, just buy regular garlic and chop it yourself.)

PANTRY SHELF STAND-BYS

Sauces

Pick your favorites: Spaghetti sauce (look for 500 mg of sodium or less per ½ cup), which also can double as pizza sauce in pita pizzas, and salsa are excellent sources of the powerful antioxidant lycopene; sweet and sour sauce makes for a low-sodium stir-fry sauce; BBQ sauce adds low-fat pizzazz to grilled food.

Serious Cereal

Make a sizable dent in your daily fiber requirement with cereals that offer at least 4 g fiber and no more than 5 g sugar or 1 g saturated fat per 100 calories. Have about 160 to 190 calories of cereal in the morning.

For the best hot cereals, go for oatmeal, multigrain, brown rice, and Wheatena—any brand whose ingredient list cites whole grains or bran. If you like to shop at natural food stores, try cereals like amaranth and quinoa. The nutritional payoff: B vitamins, fiber, minerals, and beneficial phytonutrients. There might be a weight-loss payoff too: Studies show that oatmeal (the base of many of these cereals) keeps blood sugar stable, which suppresses appetite. Bolster calcium by using equal parts fat-free or 1% milk and water or all milk instead of all water. Impart a creamier consistency by letting the grain and the liquid warm up together, instead of stirring the grain into the hot liquid. Cook with apples, bananas, or dried fruit, and top with 2 tablespoons of almonds, pecans, or other nuts of your choice.

For help on choosing a great cereal, see page 183.

Canned Beans (Legumes)

All beans are nutrient-rich, starring iron, fiber, and heart disease-fighting folic acid. White beans, navy beans (which are white!), and Great

Northern beans are good sources of calcium, offering 13 to 16 percent of the daily value per cup cooked or canned. Some brands of canned beans may have more sodium than you want. But you can substantially cut the sodium by rinsing them in running water for about a minute. There are also lower-sodium brands with less than 150 mg sodium per ½ cup that are sold in health food stores and some supermarkets. Or, if you're so inclined, you can soak dry beans overnight (or for at least 6 hours) and boil them for ½ hour for lima beans and up to 3 hours for tougher beans. You can also prepare a large batch and then freeze it in smaller amounts.

Since beans are rich in both protein and carbs, they're practically a complete meal in themselves. Dress up plain canned beans with a vinaigrette and some vegetables and you've got a meal. Or, open a can of vegetarian chili, pair it with a slice of cornbread and a vegetable for another quick, satisfying, balanced meal.

Super Tip ➤ Making Beans a "Complete" Protein

In this protein-obsessed diet culture, you might wonder whether the bean-based vegetarian meals in this book provide enough protein. It's true that protein in eggs, milk, beef, and other animal sources is "complete," i.e., composed of all the amino acids our bodies need to grow and thrive. Protein in beans—garbanzos, white beans, black beans, and the like—is "incomplete," meaning it's missing one or two crucial amino acids. However, bread and rice are flush with the very same amino acids that beans lack. (And these starches are poor in the amino acids plentiful in beans.) So, together they complement each other and give your body all the amino acids it needs. You don't have to eat beans and grains at the same meal, just on the same day. Beans are a fabulous source of fiber as well as protein. So do yourself a favor and go veggie once in a while: Vegetable protein appears to be more protective against cancer, heart disease, and other chronic diseases than animal protein.

Best Soups and Broths

The right soup can be transformed into an instant healthy and delicious meal. Stock up on lentil or other bean soups. Try the creamy—but not fatty—vegetable-based broccoli, butternut squash, portobello mushroom, or tomato soups sold in resealable paper cartons by Imagine, Pacific or Whole Foods. You'll find recipes to enhance these soups in chapter 4.

Chicken broth is a virtually fat-free way to add depth to grain pilafs, create a lean substitute for gravy, or help you make a homemade soup. Pour in just enough to barely cover vegetables, then simmer until tender, and the vegetables will taste like they've been braised in butter with none of the calories and fat. Use broths marked "low sodium" or "reduced sodium" whether in cans, aseptic cartons, or bouillon cubes.

Chicken in Cans or Pouches

Sounds a little retro, but these shelf-stable products are actually pretty good when mixed into a chicken salad, pasta sauce, or casserole. Plus, they're lower in sodium and preservatives than many refrigerated deli meats. Chicken in cans or pouches looks a lot like canned white tuna—it's firm but easily flaked. Canned chicken is packed in a little water; the meat in pouches needs no draining.

Fish in Cans or Pouches

A can of light tuna (which has lower levels of mercury than white albacore tuna) becomes a quick sandwich filler and can also be tossed with pasta or rice. Look for tuna in pouches, which may have a slightly firmer consistency and comes in a variety of flavors. Sardines are rich in healthy omega-3 fats. Try Bela Olhão brand, which is less pungent.

Great Grains

Fastest whole grains to prepare: whole-wheat couscous (8 minutes) or 90-second microwavable brown rice (such as Uncle Ben's Ready Rice). Have 15 to 25 minutes? Go for whole-wheat pasta (the Italian imports taste best), or bulgur wheat; both have a low glycemic index, meaning they don't trigger blood sugar spikes and dips.

Best Canned Vegetables

Canned tomatoes offer loads of the antioxidant lycopene; reduced-sodium varieties are also available. Pair with a can of beans, a little olive oil, and garlic, and you've got an incredibly healthy meal. Vacuum-packed, no-sodium-added corn tastes remarkably fresh; ½ cup counts as a starch serving, equivalent to a slice of bread. Always buy plain canned vegetables; avoid those packed in calorie-hiking sauces and syrups.

Best Oils

You need only stock two: olive oil (rich in heart-healthy monounsaturated fat) and canola oil (ditto for the mono, plus it's a good source of a type of plant omega-3 fatty acid). If you don't use oil within a month or if your kitchen is hot, refrigerate it. Any cloudiness or crystals will quickly disappear when you bring the oil back to room temp.

Vinegars

Have a blast experimenting with different types, each with unique charms. Balsamic is flavorful, its vinegary edge tempered by its sweetness. Raspberry and other fruit-infused vinegars go gorgeously with salads that include berries, citrus, or other fruit. Rice wine vinegar is a natural in Asian dressings (along with dark toasted sesame oil, garlic, and ginger). Seasoned rice wine vinegar can serve as a dressing all by itself! Apple cider vinegar is great for milder dressings, and various red and white wine vinegars are classic components in mustardy vinaigrettes as well as many other salad dressings and marinades, and can even be used to cut the amount of oil in sautéed vegetables.

Nuts and Nut Butters

They're all good for you: Walnuts are particularly rich in omega-3 fatty acids; almonds, cashews, peanuts, and pecans are packed with mono-unsaturated fat—another heart-healthy fat.

Dried Fruit

As you move into the winter months and juicy peaches become a wistful memory, the produce aisle might not look so inspiring. But look again, this time at the dried-fruit section, since many fruits retain much

Super Tip ➤ Vinegar

There's a secret weight-loss weapon in your pantry: vinegar. Adding vinegar to a meal lowers the "glycemic index." The glycemic index measures how quickly a food—or meal—causes blood sugar to rise. The lower the number the smaller the blood sugar spike and the less fluctuation in appetite. Research at Arizona State University, East Mesa, Arizona, found that taking 2 tablespoons of vinegar twice daily caused people to lose 2 pounds in four weeks compared to no weight loss in a placebo group getting the same amount of cranberry juice (nothing magical about cranberry juice; it's just the liquid the scientists decided to test against vinegar). Four tablespoons of vinegar daily is a little much; it's yet to be determined whether less will do. Any vinegar will work: apple cider, balsamic, raspberry, etc.

of their nutrition after drying. Cranberries and prunes are especially phytonutrient rich; dried figs are loaded with fiber; and just 2 tablespoons of chopped dried apricots supply half of the daily requirement for vitamin A. (Some dried fruit, such as mango and pineapple, has extra sugar added, so be sure to read the labels and opt for the fruit without added sugar.)

Case in point: cranberries, one of the highest sources of proanthocyanidins, powerful antioxidants that also help prevent urinary tract infections. An ounce and a half (⅓ cup dried cranberries) daily confers the same urinary tract protection as the recommended 10 ounces of cranberry juice. Unless you need that extra protection, stick to 3 tablespoons, the calorie equivalent of a piece of fruit. Dried plums (formerly known as prunes) also score high in antioxidants and are a good source of fiber.

Hot Drinks.

For just 120 calories, a 12-ounce skim-milk latte supplies 35 percent of the day's calcium recommendation (29 percent for women over age fifty,

Super Tip ➤ The Nutty Benefits

Almonds, cashews, peanuts, pecans, walnuts—take your pick; they're all good for you. Many of *The Supermarket Diet* breakfasts include a sprinkling of nuts because they help suppress your appetite and they're a heart-healthy food. Two Harvard University studies tracking the diets and health of thousands of men and women found that people who ate the most nuts had the lowest risk of heart disease or fatal heart attacks. Fortunately, you don't have to eat lots of nuts to get the protective effect since nuts are high in calories. In the women's study (Nurses Health Study), eating just an ounce of nuts (a scant 1/4 cup) five or more times per week was linked to a 35 percent reduced risk for heart disease.

Here's why nuts are so protective. They are:

▶ Rich in alpha-linolenic acid, a type of omega-3 fatty acid that partially converts to one of the heart-protective omega-3 fatty acids in fish. Best sources: pine nuts and walnuts.

▶ High in monounsaturated fat, which helps lower cholesterol. In several research studies, diets supplemented with nuts caused a drop in blood cholesterol. Best sources: almonds, hazelnuts, peanuts, pine nuts, and pistachios.

▶ Nutrient rich. Nuts are good sources of the following nutrients, all essential for normal heart function: folic acid (especially peanuts), magnesium (especially almonds), potassium (especially pistachios), and vitamin E (especially hazelnuts and almonds). Brazil nuts are a phenomenal source of selenium, a mineral that helps prevent cancer.

▶ Rich in arginine. This amino acid is a building block of nitric oxide, a compound that relaxes arteries and lowers blood pressure. Best sources: peanuts, pecans, and pine nuts.

who have a higher calcium requirement). Polyphenols in black and green tea have been linked to lower risk of heart disease, and if you prefer to avoid caffeine, herbal teas are a calorie-free way to relax.

Spice Staples

Curry lovers, take note: Turmeric, the base of curry powder, contains curcumin, a powerful antioxidant shown to prevent cancer in lab animals. Other antioxidant superstars: allspice, cinnamon (just ½ teaspoon of cinnamon daily helps lower blood sugar), clove, garlic powder, ginger, oregano, pepper, peppermint, and sage. Stock up on your favorites to season chicken and tuna salads, marinades, pasta dishes, salad dressing, and more.

Throw 'Em Out!

Just as a sensibly stocked kitchen will help you lose weight, having too many fattening foods on hand will undermine your weight-loss effort. The safest way to deal with sweets, chips, and other tempting foods is the "one-treat rule": Keep *just one portion* of *just one treat* around the house. No boxes of cookies or big bags of chips; buy the single-portion packets one at a time instead. On the Keep On Losin' plan you get a daily 125-calorie snack. That number—or something close to it—should be the calorie count of your treat. Nabisco, for instance, has packaged 100 calories worth of crackers and other snacks. Read labels carefully to get those lowest in trans fat.

If you've got to cater to family members who insist on having their junk food, then keep it out of your sight and avoid any temptation. Have them hide it from you, if possible, or put it all in one cupboard or in a big Tupperware container in the fridge. (They can even lock the cupboard if necessary!)

Now, check out this list and start throwing out your diet busters! These are items you don't need hanging around tempting you:

FREEZER FOES

- *Ice cream.* Better not to stock ice cream at all, but if you must, keep only one little something (125 calories or less) in there at a time.

Anything bigger than a *single* Snickers ice cream bar or just *one* Good Humor bar or a little 4-ounce cup of Italian ice is potential trouble. Can you really stop at just 4 tablespoons of Häagen Dazs (135 calories)? Can you really eat just one Skinny Cow Silhouette ice cream sandwich and leave the rest of the six-pack alone? A good option is light ice cream or frozen yogurt: With about 110 calories per half cup, it gives you a decent-sized portion for the calories. You can also make this convenience food *inconvenient* by not keeping it on hand. Then when you really want it, you have to motivate yourself to go to your local convenience store or market, and even then, you will get only one bar.

- *Frozen cakes, pies, pastries, cookies, etc.* Same deal as the ice cream: Get rid of anything that's bigger than a small cookie or sliver of pound cake. And stick to the "one sweet" rule: If you've got ice cream, don't keep any other sweets on hand.
- *High-calorie dinners.* That frozen mac 'n' cheese or fried chicken dinner with a zillion fat grams was your stress buddy, but it's time to evict him along with any other frozen dinner that exceeds 450 calories. (But go ahead and try the Healthy Choice and Lean Cuisine mac 'n' cheese dinners. Just add lots of vegetables.)

REFRIGERATOR REJECTS

- *Whole or 2% milk.* Wean yourself down slowly to 1% or fat free; the extra calories and fat grams are better spent elsewhere. If you really like a fuller-bodied milk in your coffee, keep a half-pint of 2% or half-and-half just for that purpose only. Or try whipping up fat-free or 1% with a little hand-held whipper; it takes only seconds to make the milk thick and creamy. A tablespoon of 2% milk is just 7 calories; no need to count it unless you're taking in more than 4 tablespoons daily. But each tablespoon of half-and-half is 20 calories; any more than that should be drawn from your treat account.
- *White-flour biscuits, rolls, croissants, pop-and-heat pastries, etc.* Chuck 'em all. Stick with whole-grain breads which make you feel fuller for longer than white-flour products.
- *Pudding or other sweets.* Your M.O.: the "one sweet" rule. Sugar-free puddings are 60 to 90 calories per single-serving container (3 to 4 ounces), which make a much smaller dent in your 125-calorie treat allowance than the 160 calories for regular.

- *Regular mayo.* Cut the fat in mayo with low-fat plain yogurt in recipes, but since reduced-fat mayo tastes so good *and* you can even dilute calories further by cutting with yogurt, why not make it your staple?
- *Onion dip or other high-fat dips.* If you can relegate them to your 125-calorie treats, keep them; otherwise, toss.
- *Hot dogs.* The ultimate junk food. You're getting anywhere from about 150 to 250 calories per wiener, most of which is fat, and, even worse, most of that is artery-clogging saturated fat! If you've just gotta have one on occasion, get the reduced-fat or soy versions.

PANTRY PURGING

- *Box of cookies.* Yes, it's impossible to buy a single Oreo. So, if the unbearable craving strikes, go to the drugstore and buy a six-pack. Or, go to the bakery and buy two little cookies, or even one medium-to-big cookie (skip the ones as big as your face, please!). Or, if you won't eat more than one bag of 100-calorie Nabisco treats, stock these. This strategy means you'll never go through an entire box to console yourself, then hate yourself the next day. And yes, you're still following the "one sweet" policy. A cookie in the pantry means no sweets in the fridge or freezer!
- *Fiber-poor cereal or granola.* Some brands of cornflakes may be light in calories compared to some other cereals, but since they're so fiber-poor, they have no staying power. You're hungry an hour later. And granola is so high calorie, you've reached your calorie quota with just a quarter cup. So, stick with the cereal guidelines in the "Foods to Have on Hand" section.
- *Chips, cheese puffs, pretzels, and other salty snacks.* Treat these as you would sweets and cookies: If buying a big bag means eating much more than your daily treat allowance (125 calories on the Keep On Losin' plan), then get rid of the bag. Safer to keep a 1-ounce bag, which runs about 140 to 150 calories for regular and 110 to 130 for the baked versions.
- *Ramen noodles.* A serving is nearly a meal's worth of calories (about 300), and all you get is fat, white-flour carbs, and more than half the day's sodium allotment. Move on to whole-grain pastas.

3 Pound-Paring Boot Camp

Whether you've got 10 pounds to lose or 200, dropping those first few pounds is pretty darn exciting. You can ride that momentum to drop the next few pounds and the next and the next . . . That's what these first two weeks of boot camp are all about: a pound-peeling, motivating jump start. At 1,200 calories a day plus exercise, you'll soon see results on your scale. (Start the exercise plan in chapter 5 the day you start the Boot Camp meal plan or sooner!) But unlike a crazy fad diet that you can barely stand for two weeks, you'll be eating normal food you like, easily purchased at your supermarket. This plan is setting you up for a lifetime of weight control: Both the Boot Camp and Keep On Losin' plans teach you lifelong eating and exercise habits. Note to men: skip Boot Camp—the calories are too low—and go straight to the Keep On Losin' plan, chapter 4.

But *boot camp*? Don't worry, this won't be punishing; that wouldn't be very inspiring! You'll simply be eating 300 calories less per day than on the rest of *The Supermarket Diet*. You might lose 5 pounds, maybe less, but you *will* shed some fat if you follow the Boot Camp prescription. Plus, you'll feel better, lighter, and more energetic.

The reason Boot Camp lasts just two weeks is that your metabolism will slow down, slowing down your long-term weight loss, if you go on such a low-calorie diet for a prolonged period of time. Use these two weeks to jump-start your weight loss, then move on to Keep On Losin', a 1,500-calorie plan. If after two days Boot Camp feels too restrictive and you find that you're hungry all the time, switch immediately to Keep On Losin'.

The next two weeks are completely mapped out for you. All you have to do is show up and follow the plan. To make this as fail-proof as possible, *The Supermarket Diet* Boot Camp gives you:

- shopping lists
- a list of foods to avoid (just for two weeks)
- quick, easy-to-prepare meals
- an exercise program (see chapter 5)

Ready? C'mon. Let's go shopping!

Boot Camp Shopping Lists

These lists at first may look like a ton of food, but you'll be using the food over the course of the weeks ahead. The lists assume you have *nothing* in your kitchen, not even salt! So, go through and scratch off the foods you already have. (For your convenience, you will find printable copies of the shopping list on *Good Housekeeping*'s website:

Eating with the Family

You can easily feed the rest of your family any of the meals in *The Supermarket Diet.* This isn't "diet food" but normal food in moderate portions. Family members can simply enjoy larger portions. For instance, on the first day of Boot Camp, your teenage son can have two chicken wraps for lunch, while you have one. Your husband can add more pecans and dressing to the Spinach Salad for dinner, have more crackers, and perhaps finish with a piece of fruit. Many of *The Supermarket Diet* recipes—for Boot Camp, Keep On Losin', and Stay Slim Maintenance—serve four or six people. Take out your calorie-controlled serving, then let the rest of the family have as much as they like!

Go to www.goodhousekeeping.com). There are no portions on the shopping list, as the quantities you buy will depend on the number of people in your family. So, just go through the menu plan and note how much of everything you'll need.

Week One ➤ Shopping List

For some fresh foods you'll find notes about the day of the week they're needed so that you don't buy them too far ahead of time. You may also want to consult the Boot Camp Recipes starting on page 53 so that you can see exactly when all the foods are required.

FRESH PRODUCE
Fruits

☐ Apples
☐ Bananas
☐ Blueberries
☐ Cantaloupe (optional)
☐ Grapes
☐ Lemons

☐ Limes
☐ Mangoes
☐ Oranges
☐ Raspberries (optional)
☐ Strawberries (or get frozen)
☐ Tangerines (or oranges)

Vegetables/Herbs

☐ Asparagus
☐ Avocado
☐ Broccoli
☐ Carrots, baby
☐ Cauliflower (optional)
☐ Celery
☐ Cilantro
☐ Garlic
☐ Lettuce, romaine or butterhead

☐ Mixed greens
☐ Onions, red
☐ Onions, white
☐ Parsley
☐ Pepper, red
☐ Spinach
☐ Tomatoes
☐ Watercress

Beans, Soup, Tuna and Vegetables

- ☐ Refried beans, canned, 100 to 140 calories and under 500 mg sodium per 1/2 cup, such as Old El Paso Vegetarian Refried Beans or Amy's Organic Traditional Refried Beans
- ☐ Soup, lentil, 130 to 150 calories and under 600 mg sodium per cup, such as Progresso Lentil 99% fat-free (it's lower in sodium than the regular Progresso Lentil) or Amy's Light in Sodium Organic Lentil Vegetable. Or, go to the frozen foods section and get Tabatchnick Lentil Soup.

- ☐ Tomatoes in puree, canned whole (if unavailable, use whole tomatoes in juice), preferably reduced-sodium, such as Hunt's Whole Tomatoes, no sodium added (if making single serving of the Penne Rigate, get marinara sauce instead)
- ☐ Tuna, chunk-light, in water (or in pouch)

Dressings and Condiments

- ☐ Dressing, ranch, light, 70 to 80 calories per 2 tablespoons, such as Annie's Naturals Organic Buttermilk Dressing, Hidden Valley Lite or Kraft Light Done Right. For variety, get two of your favorites in this same calorie range.
- ☐ Jalapeño chiles, pickled (optional)
- ☐ Ketchup
- ☐ Mango chutney
- ☐ Mayonnaise, reduced-fat, 45 to 50 calories per tablespoon, such as Hellmann's Light or Kraft Light

- ☐ Mustard
- ☐ Olive oil
- ☐ Olives, salad olives or pimiento-stuffed green olives (1/4 cup)
- ☐ Salsa, no more than 150 mg sodium per 2 tablespoons, such as Chi Chi's Fiesta Salsa Thick and Chunky, or any of the Newman's Own Salsas (Newman's Own Peach Salsa is especially delicious!)
- ☐ Vinegar

Drinks

- ☐ Beer, light or nonalcoholic
- ☐ Coffee, regular or decaf
- ☐ V-8 juice (optional)

Spreads

- ☐ Honey
- ☐ Jam or jelly
- ☐ Nut butter (peanut or almond), such as Smuckers Peanut Butter or 365 (Whole Foods label) Almond Butter

DRY GOODS/BREAD

Breads

- ☐ Bread, 100% whole-wheat
- ☐ Burger buns, whole-wheat, 115 to 130 calories. If you can't find these, get sourdough rolls.
- ☐ Pitas, whole-wheat

Cereal

- ☐ High-fiber cereal with at least 4 g fiber per 100 calories (or 6 g per 150 calories) and preferably no more than 5 g sugar per 100 calories (8 g per 150 calories), such as All-Bran Extra Fiber, Fiber 1; Kashi GoLean (not GoLean Crunch); Kellogg's Complete Oat Bran Flakes. Some brands of raisin bran are also OK, but they may be higher in sugar because of the raisins. Look for lower-sugar brands such as Health Valley or 365 (Whole Foods label).

Crackers

- ☐ Crackers, whole-grain, such as Ak Mak, RyKrisp, or Triscuit

Dried Fruit

- ☐ Raisins, dark, seedless

Dried Spices

☐ Cinnamon

☐ Curry powder

☐ Garlic powder

☐ Pepper, black

☐ Pepper, ground red (cayenne)

☐ Salt

Energy bars

☐ "Energy" bar with 220 to 240 calories and at least 4 g fiber. Odwalla Carrot Bar, Power Bar Harvest (not dipped), or Clif bar are good choices.

Nuts

☐ Pecans, unsalted

☐ Walnuts or other unsalted nuts

Pasta

☐ Pasta, whole wheat (bow-ties, penne rigate, ziti, or other short, tubular pasta), such as Ronzoni Healthy Harvest penne rigate or Bionaturae whole durum wheat pastas (available at Whole Foods)

REFRIGERATED SECTIONS

Dairy and Eggs

☐ Cheese, feta (crumbled or solid)

☐ Cheese, reduced-fat, such as Cabot 50% Cheddar or Kraft 2% singles

☐ Eggs

☐ Lemon juice (or, even better, freshly squeezed)

☐ Milk, fat-free (needed often throughout the week)

☐ Tortillas, flour, 8-inch, 120 to 130 calories, preferably whole-wheat or fiber-enriched, such as 365 Organic Whole Wheat Tortillas (Whole Foods label) or La Tortilla Factory 99% Fat-Free burrito size

☐ Yogurt, plain low-fat, such as Dannon Plain Lowfat or Stonyfield Farms Organic Lowfat

Meat/Poultry/Fish

- ☐ Beef, ground, 90% lean
- ☐ Chicken, rotisserie, about 2 pounds (for use on Sunday, so buy on Saturday or Sunday)
- ☐ Chicken breast (for use on Monday)
- ☐ Salmon steaks, 1 inch thick, 4 ounces each (for use on Saturday, so buy on Friday or Saturday)
- ☐ turkey breast, sliced (for use on Thursday)

Frozen Foods

- ☐ Breakfast Burrito, Amy's brand (if not preparing your own)
- ☐ Burgers, soy-based vegetable (Boca All-American Flame Grilled or Gardenburger Flame Grilled are soy-based, meaning soy is the first or second ingredient.)
- ☐ Fruit juice bar, no more than 70 calories
- ☐ Microwavable meal, 400 to 420 calories with at least 5 g fiber and no more than 3 g saturated fat. Some of the best-tasting and nutritious frozen meals are ethnic (Indian, Mexican, Asian). Look for brand names such as Amy's and Taj (both found in supermarkets and health food stores) as well as more widely known names like Lean Cuisine and Healthy Choice.
- ☐ Pizza, vegetarian, 380 calories, such as DiGiorno Pizza Rising Crust Vegetable Pizza, any of the Lean Cuisine Café Classics pizzas, any of the Amy's pizzas
- ☐ Soup, lentil, Tabatchnick brand (if not buying canned soup)
- ☐ Strawberries (or fresh, if you prefer)

Week Two ➤ Shopping List

You have some foods for week two left over from week one's shopping trip. Here are the rest of the provisions you'll need to stock up on. However, you may need to restock some week one items if more than one family member is following the diet. Take a look at the menus for week two to make sure you have what you need.

FRESH PRODUCE

Fruits

- ☐ Apples
- ☐ Bananas
- ☐ Blueberries
- ☐ Grapes
- ☐ Limes
- ☐ Oranges
- ☐ Strawberries (or use frozen)

Vegetables/Herbs

- ☐ Vegetables, bag of fresh-cut mixed (broccoli, carrots, snap peas, celery blend)
- ☐ Broccoli (or use frozen)
- ☐ Butternut squash (if making Butternut Soup from scratch; otherwise skip this, and buy a ready-made soup)
- ☐ Cucumbers (optional)
- ☐ Corn-on-the-cob
- ☐ Dill, fresh (optional)
- ☐ Garlic
- ☐ Ginger, fresh
- ☐ Green onions
- ☐ Greens, mustard, or red or Swiss chard
- ☐ Jalapeño peppers
- ☐ Lettuce, romaine or butterhead
- ☐ Mixed greens
- ☐ Onions
- ☐ Parsley (optional)
- ☐ Peppers, red
- ☐ Snow peas
- ☐ Spinach
- ☐ Tomatoes
- ☐ Zucchini

Dressings and Condiments

- ☐ Canola oil
- ☐ Horseradish (optional)
- ☐ Maple syrup
- ☐ Stir-fry sauce
- ☐ Teriyaki sauce

Beans and Soup

- ☐ Chicken broth, preferably reduced-sodium, such as Campbell's Low-Sodium Chicken Broth and Pacific Low-Sodium Organic Chicken Broth
- ☐ Soup, black bean, preferably under 600 mg sodium per cup, such as Progresso or Amy's Black Bean Vegetable
- ☐ Soup, butternut squash (if not making from scratch), preferably under 600 mg sodium per cup, such as Amy's Light in Sodium Butternut Squash Soup, or Pacific Creamy Butternut Squash Soup

Other

- ☐ Chocolate syrup, such as Hershey's syrup, about 50 calories per tablespoon.
- ☐ Marinara sauce, preferably under 600 mg sodium per 1/2 cup, such as Bertolli or Newman's Own
- ☐ Pineapple chunks in juice, such as Dole 100% Natural Pineapple Chunks in Juice

DRY GOODS/BREAD
Breads

- ☐ Bread, 100% whole-wheat
- ☐ Pitas, whole-wheat

Cereal

☐ High-fiber cereal with at least 4 g fiber per 100 calories (or 6 g per 150 calories) and preferably no more than 5 g sugar per 100 calories (8 g per 150 calories), such as All-Bran Extra Fiber, Fiber 1; Kashi GoLean (not GoLean Crunch); Kellogg's Complete Oat Bran Flakes. Some brands of raisin bran are also OK, but they may be higher in sugar than these others because of the raisins. Look for lower-sugar brands such as Health Valley or 365 (Whole Foods label).

☐ Oatmeal. Opt for Quaker Oats or any other brand of plain oatmeal over the instant or preflavored varieties. If you have time to cook, try steel-cut oats, such as McCann's Steel Cut Irish Oatmeal.

Dried Spices

☐ Hot pepper flakes
☐ Oregano, dried

☐ Paprika

Nuts

☐ Almonds or walnuts

Rice/Pasta

☐ Couscous, preferably whole-wheat, such as Fantastic Foods Organic Whole Wheat Couscous
☐ Pasta, whole-wheat (spaghetti, penne, or other pasta of your choice), such as Ronzoni Healthy Harvest penne rigate or Bionaturae Whole Durum Wheat Pastas (available at Whole Foods)

☐ Rice, brown, regular or instant, such as Uncle Ben's Whole-Grain Brown Ready Rice

Sugar/Flour

- ☐ Cornmeal, yellow
- ☐ Cornstarch
- ☐ Flour, all-purpose
- ☐ Sugar, brown

Dairy and Eggs

- ☐ Cheese, reduced-fat (feta, Swiss, or Cheddar)
- ☐ Milk, fat-free (needed often throughout the week)
- ☐ Yogurt, flavored low-fat
- ☐ Yogurt, plain low-fat, such as Dannon Plain Lowfat or Stonyfield Farms Organic Lowfat Plain Yogurt

Spreads

- ☐ Hummus (or make your own)
- ☐ Margarine, trans fat–free, 70 to 80 calories per tablespoon, such as Fleischmann's Made with Olive Oil, or Smart Balance 67% Buttery Spread

Meat/Poultry/Fish

Some of these foods are needed in the middle or end of the week, so don't buy them at the beginning of the week. Check recipes starting on page 53 to determine when you want to buy them.

- ☐ Beef, ground, 95% lean
- ☐ Chicken, rotisserie
- ☐ Chicken, white-meat, cooked
- ☐ Pork tenderloin (or skinless chicken breast)
- ☐ Roast beef, sliced, lean, such as Healthy Choice or Boar's Head (for use on Saturday, so buy on Friday or Saturday)
- ☐ Trout, brook or rainbow (1/4 pound each)

Frozen Foods

- ☐ Berries (if fresh are unavailable)
- ☐ Broccoli (if fresh is unavailable)
- ☐ Shrimp, large, shelled and deveined

Boot Camp Chow

Welcome to a very slimming 1,200-calorie-per-day eating plan. These meals are crammed with fruits, vegetables, and other low-cal-but-filling foods. For the best results don't forget to lace up your sneakers and get moving. Although this plan is nutritionally balanced, it's impossible to get every last milligram of every vitamin and mineral on just 1,200 calories. So, over the next two weeks of Boot Camp, supplement your food with a multi-vitamin/mineral tablet. Get a multi with about 100 percent of the Daily Value (DV) for all vitamins and minerals (the standard levels set by the Food and Drug Administration); avoid those that douse you with high levels or make you take more than one tablet. For instance, Centrum or Centrum Silver for those over age fifty are good choices. If you're over age fifty, take a 200 to 500 mg calcium supplement as well.

Remember that men should skip Boot Camp and go straight to Keep On Losin'.

SWAPPING FOOD ON THE PLAN

Follow this plan as closely as possible. You should not swap one breakfast for another breakfast, or one lunch or dinner for another lunch or dinner. That's because these meals vary in calories; breakfast on one day could be 100 calories higher than on another. The plan is structured this way so that you can indulge a little: For instance, have a pizza, salad, and beer dinner balanced by a breakfast and lunch that are modest in calories. In the upcoming 1,500-calorie plan, like meals are equal in calories (i.e. all the breakfasts are the same number of calories, the lunches the same, the dinners and snacks the same). So, in two weeks, you can meal-swap all you like.

It's OK to make some changes just as long as you don't increase or decrease the calorie level and the basic meal composition. That means eating the same amounts of dairy, fat, fruits, proteins, and vegetables that are in these meals. For instance, you can substitute 3 ounces of tofu or shrimp for 3 ounces of chicken or lean meat. You can have a cup of Brussels sprouts instead of a cup of broccoli. If you're in too much of a hurry to make pasta or rice, swap 1 slice of whole-wheat bread for every half cup of cooked pasta or cooked rice. A teaspoon of trans fat–free margarine can take the place of a teaspoon of olive oil. Take note: The bread in this plan should be no more than 65 to 75 calories per slice, so read labels carefully.

Whatever you do, don't skip a meal! That will set you up for overeating later.

FEELING HUNGRY?

Give your stomach a few days to shrink before you decide that Boot Camp is not for you. But if you're following the plan to the "T" and still feeling hungry much of the day after the first three days, try adding another 100 calories daily. Here are a few examples of 100 calories' worth of food:

Beans, black or garbanzo, or any other type of legume, 1/3 cup
Bread, preferably whole-wheat, 1¹/2 slices
Broccoli, 4 cups cooked
Cheese, 2 slices 2% singles, or 1¹/2 ounces reduced-fat Cheddar or Swiss (check label to make sure)
Chicken, grilled, 2 ounces (2/3 the size of a deck of cards)
Greens, mixed, 2¹/2 cups, with a salad dressing containing 2 teaspoons olive oil
Milk, fat-free, 1¹/4 cups
Nuts, 2 tablespoons (about 15 almonds, about 18 cashews or peanuts),
Oil, olive, canola, or other, 2¹/2 teaspoons
Rice or pasta (plain), 1/2 cup cooked
Sweet potato, 1 medium (2 inches in diameter, 5 inches in length)
Turkey breast, deli-sliced, 3 ounces

If after another two days you're still feeling deprived, then skip the rest of Boot Camp. Instead, start the Keep On Losin' Plan in chapter 3. That plan is 1,500 calories, still low enough to produce about a pound of weight loss per week, perhaps even more.

Keep Yourself Honest:
The Food Diary

If Boot Camp isn't working, i.e., you're not losing weight or you feel out-of-control and are overeating, you need to quickly figure out what's going wrong. Your sleuth: a food journal. By writing down everything you're eating, you'll see how you're diverging from the plan. Perhaps you skipped a meal and felt justified overeating (and having dessert) at the next one. Or you had a beer, then another one!

You will detect not only the diet culprits but also the triggers. The Food Diary (appendix 3, page 269) has an entry for "Time/Place" and another entry for "Emotions/Situation." You might discover that most of your overeating occurs in the kitchen while you're on the phone (that's my guilty spot) or that those vending-machine snacks happen when "Bored at work" is scribbled in the "Emotions/Situation" entry.

Use the Food Diary as needed throughout your weight loss—and weight maintenance—to keep you on track.

FILLING OUT A FOOD JOURNAL

To get the most accurate picture of your diet, record your intake as accurately as possible. There's no such thing as being too obsessive. It's a good idea to measure the foods that you eat regularly at least once so that you can record them accurately. For instance, pour out your usual bowl of cereal, or portion of rice, etc. Then, measure the portion and figure out the calories from the nutrition facts label. Here are some general guidelines to help you get the most out of the journal.

- Write down *every* morsel you take in, even if it's just two M&Ms.
- Be specific: Was it 1% or skim milk? Whole-wheat bread or white? Did the tuna salad have a lot of mayonnaise or was it dry? A packet of sugar in the latte? And how large was that latte?
- Record all beverages, including water and alcohol, and specify amounts in ounces or cups. The reason to record water, even though it's calorie-free, is to get a sense of your fluid intake. Sometimes you can mistake thirst for hunger, so it's important to get enough fluid.

- Be sure to record hunger levels: Hunger level 1 = full; 2 = not hungry, not full; 3 = hungry; 4 = very hungry; 5 = desperately hungry. Ideally, you should be eating at a 3, sometimes a 4. Otherwise you're eating when you're not hungry (a 1 or a 2) or when you're so hungry you're at risk for overeating (a 5).
- Under "Emotions," scribble down anything you think might be relevant ("responding to a craving," "super-stressed at work," etc.) You don't have to fill this out each time, just when it seems useful. This way, you start making links between food and emotions.
- Save nutrition labels on foods to help you add up calories. Even better, jot down fiber along with calories to get a daily tally of this diet friend.
- Write down the details of your meals as soon as possible after eating. Research shows that people tend to get less accurate the longer they wait to record.

Boot Camp No-No List

To get results, stick very closely to the plan. If you're tempted to stray during these two weeks, don't eat any of the following. They'll send calories soaring and knock you off the plan. (Don't worry, we'll bring back some of these foods in the Keep On Losin' part of the program):

▶ All deep-fried food. Examples: French fries, onion rings, fried chicken.
▶ Any caloric beverage except those specified on this plan: fat-free milk and the occasional light beer. Drink water, and a diet drink or two a day is fine. But you need to avoid fruit juice, soda pop, beer, and sugared iced teas.
▶ Don't use more than 1 teaspoon of sugar in your coffee or tea.
▶ Other than the two breakfast smoothies offered on the plan, stay away from smoothies during the rest of Boot Camp. While they can be healthy, they are high calorie and serve as a complete meal.

Please record at least five days: ideally, three workdays and one weekend. Five days, especially five consecutive days, give a good picture of your diet. We have provided you with five days' worth of diary pages. You can copy the page for future diaries or you can download them from *Good Housekeeping*'s website at www.goodhousekeeping.com

1 Week One ➤ Boot Camp Menus at a Glance

These days average 1,200 calories. You get about 25 g fiber a day, nice and high to facilitate weight loss. Sodium averages 1,750 mg daily, well below the 2,300 cap currently recommended by the government, to help reduce bloat and lower blood pressure.

MONDAY (page 54)

Breakfast	Lunch	Snack	Dinner
Cereal, fruit, and nuts Milk	Chicken Wrap Baby carrots and red pepper	Skim latte	Spinach Salad with Eggs, Orange, and Pecans Whole-grain crackers

TUESDAY (page 54)

Breakfast	Lunch	Snack	Dinner
Power bar Milk	Tuna Salad Sandwich Red pepper or V-8 juice	Grapes	Penne Rigate with Sweet-and-Spicy Picadillo Sauce Asparagus

WEDNESDAY (page 58)

Breakfast	Snack	Lunch	Dinner
Cinnamon-Apple Peanut Butter Toast Milk	Grapes	Penne Rigate with Sweet-and-Spicy Picadillo Sauce	Greek Lentil Soup Whole-wheat pita

THURSDAY (page 58)

Breakfast	Lunch	Dinner	Snack
Cereal, fruit, and nuts Milk	Turkey and Swiss Sandwich Salad	Microwavable meal	Frozen fruit juice bar

FRIDAY (page 60)

Breakfast	Lunch	Dinner
Smoothie Nuts	Bean Burrito	Pizza, salad, and beer!

SATURDAY (page 61)

Breakfast	Lunch	Snack	Dinner
Egg Burrito Fruit Milk or café au lait	Veggie Cheeseburger Baby carrots	Milk	Parsley Pesto Salmon Watercress Salad

SUNDAY (page 63)

Breakfast	Lunch	Dinner
Cereal, fruit, and nuts Milk	Peanut Butter and Apple Sandwich Milk Crudités	Curried Chicken and Mango Salad

2 Week Two ➤ Boot Camp Menus at a Glance

MONDAY (page 66)

Breakfast	Lunch	Snack	Dinner
Apple Oatmeal with Brown Sugar Milk	Curried Chicken and Mango Salad	Plain yogurt with nuts and honey	Shrimp and Pineapple Stir-Fry

TUESDAY (page 67)

Breakfast	Lunch	Dinner
Nut Butter and toast Milk Orange	Shrimp and Pineapple Stir-Fry	Cuban-style Black Bean Soup Bread Fruit with yogurt

WEDNESDAY (page 67)

Breakfast	Lunch	Dinner
Cereal, fruit and nuts Milk	Pita and Hummus Salad	Spaghetti with Meat Sauce Broccoli

THURSDAY (page 69)

Breakfast	Lunch	Dinner
Yogurt, fruit, and nuts	Greek Salad Whole-wheat pita	Rotisserie chicken Corn-on-the-cob Sautéed Greens

FRIDAY (page 70)

Breakfast	Lunch	Snack	Dinner
Banana	Roast-beef	Yogurt	Middle
Oatmeal with	Sandwich		Eastern
Brown sugar			Mezze
Milk			Whole-wheat
			pita

SATURDAY (page 70)

Breakfast	Lunch	Dinner
Smoothie	Chicken Salad	Asian Stir-fry
Nuts	with Grapes	Brown rice
		Light beer

SUNDAY (page 72)

Breakfast	Snack	Lunch	Dinner
Scrambled	Milk with	Butternut	Trout with
eggs, toast,	chocolate	Squash Soup	Cornmeal
and fruit	syrup	with	Crust and
		Couscous,	Spicy Corn
		Spinach, and	Relish
		Chicken	Cauliflower or
			broccoli

1 Week One ➤ Boot Camp Recipes

You'll find that some of the recipes, particularly main dishes for dinner, yield more than one portion. *The Supermarket Diet* assumes that you may be cooking for more than one person. Remember—for family members who are not on the diet, you can simply increase the size of their portions. If you find you have leftovers, simply freeze them for use after you've completed Boot Camp.

Breakfast
Cereal, fruit, and nuts: 190 calories of high-fiber cereal with ½ cup blueberries, raspberries, chopped apples, or other fruit of your choice, 2 tablespoons walnuts or other unsalted nuts, and 1 cup fat-free milk

Lunch
▶ Chicken Wrap
Loosely wrap in an *8-inch flour tortilla* (preferably whole wheat): *2 ounces cooked diced skinless chicken breast* (cook your own or use 2 refrigerated precooked slices) or a scant *½ cup strips*; *½ cup watercress; ½ slice reduced-fat cheese,* torn into smaller pieces; and *1 tablespoon light ranch dressing.*

Serve with ½ cup baby carrots and ¼ cup chopped red pepper.

Or, at Subway: Order the Chicken Bacon Ranch Wrap *without* the ranch dressing or the bacon. Substitute fat-free honey mustard dressing, and stuff with lettuce, tomato, and green pepper. Bring your own baby carrots.

Snack
12 ounces fat-free (skim) latte with sugar-free vanilla syrup, if desired.

Dinner
▶ Spinach Salad with Eggs, Orange, and Pecans
In a large salad bowl, toss together *3 cups spinach; 1 small orange (or tangerine),* peeled, seeded, and sliced; *1 to 2 tablespoons chopped red onion; 1 to 2 tablespoons light ranch or other light dressing* of your choice (or make your own with 2 teaspoons olive oil, a spritz of lemon juice, and 2 teaspoons o.j.). Top with *2 hard-cooked eggs,* cut in half, and *1 tablespoon coarsely chopped toasted pecans* (or any other type of nut).

Serve with 50 to 60 calories of whole-grain crackers, such as Triscuits, Ak Mak, or RyKrisp (check labels).

Breakfast
Power bar: 1 energy bar with 220 to 240 calories and at least 4 g fiber. Odwalla Carrot Bar is an excellent choice. Also Power Bar Harvest Bar

SuperTip ➤ Nuts—Even Peanut Butter!—*Are* Diet Food

Dieters have long viewed nuts as an enemy of their cause. Sure, nuts are high-calorie, being composed mainly of fat. But in moderation—about 2 tablespoons daily—nuts can actually help you out. By adding some fat to otherwise fat-free meals (like cereal and fat-free milk), nuts help slow down stomach emptying, making you feel fuller longer. Nuts are even more appetite-suppressing than other fats. When people spread peanut butter on their morning bagel they felt less hungry hours later than those who ate the same number of calories with a butter-spread bagel, according to research at Arizona State University, East Mesa. Nuts are also good for your heart (see page 31). Buy roasted and unsalted for big flavor without the extra sodium.

(not dipped) or a Clif bar are good choices. Have with 8 ounces fat-free milk.

Snack
½ cup grapes (about 16 grapes)

Lunch
Try the Classic, Curried or Southwestern versions of the Classic Tuna Salad recipe below. Make half the recipe and stuff between 2 slices of whole-wheat bread (with lettuce and tomato, if desired). Serve with a medium red pepper, sliced, or 6 ounces V-8 juice.

▶ Classic Tuna Salad
Prep: 15 minutes ▪ Makes 2 servings (about 1¼ cups)

1 can (6 ounces) chunk-light tuna in water, drained and flaked
   (or a 6- or 7-ounce pouch)
2 stalks celery, finely chopped
3 tablespoons reduced-fat mayonnaise
1 to 2 tablespoons low-fat, plain yogurt
2 teaspoons fresh lemon juice
1/4 teaspoon ground black pepper

In small bowl, with fork, combine tuna, celery, mayonnaise, yogurt, lemon juice, and pepper. Use enough yogurt to achieve desired consistency. Cover and refrigerate if not serving right away.
Each serving without bread: About 160 calories ■ 22 g protein ■ 5 g carbohydrate ■ 0 g fiber ■ 5 g total fat (1 g saturated) ■ 31 mg cholesterol ■ 417 mg sodium.

▶ Curried Tuna Salad
Prepare Classic Tuna Salad as above. Stir in *½ Granny Smith apple,* cored and finely chopped, and *1 teaspoon curry powder.*
Each serving without bread: About 180 calories ■ 22 g protein ■ 10 g carbohydrate ■ 1 g fiber ■ 6 g total fat (1 g saturated) ■ 31 mg cholesterol ■ 404 mg sodium.

▶ Southwestern Tuna Salad
Prepare Classic Tuna Salad as above. Stir in *2 tablespoons chopped fresh cilantro* and *1 pickled jalapeño chile,* finely chopped. Serve rolled up in warm *whole-wheat flour tortillas,* if you like.
Each serving without tortilla: About 165 calories ■ 22 g protein ■ 7 g carbohydrate ■ 1 g fiber ■ 5 g total fat (1 g saturated) ■ 31 mg cholesterol ■ 471 mg sodium.

Dinner
▶ Penne Rigate with Sweet-and-Spicy Picadillo Sauce
Have one serving and save at least one other serving for tomorrow's lunch. Or if you're serving just yourself, prepare the quick, one-portion version. Serve with 8 spears of steamed asparagus with a spritz of lemon juice.
Prep: 10 minutes ■ Cook: 15 minutes ■ Makes 6 servings

1 package (16 ounces) penne rigata, bow-tie pasta, or radiatore
   pasta, preferably whole-wheat
2 teaspoons olive oil
1 small onion, finely chopped
2 cloves garlic, crushed with garlic press
$1/4$ teaspoon ground cinnamon
$1/8$ to $1/4$ teaspoon ground red pepper (cayenne)
$3/4$ pound 90% lean ground beef
salt
1 can ($14^1/2$ ounces) whole tomatoes in puree (if unavailable,
   use whole tomatoes in juice), preferably reduced sodium
$1/2$ cup dark seedless raisins
$1/4$ cup salad olives, drained, or chopped pimiento-stuffed olives
chopped fresh parsley for garnish

1. In large saucepot, prepare pasta in boiling salted water as label
directs.

2. Meanwhile, in nonstick 12-inch skillet, heat olive oil over medium
heat until hot. Add onion and cook, stirring frequently, until tender,
about 5 minutes. Stir in garlic, cinnamon, and ground red pepper; cook
30 seconds. Increase heat to medium-high; add ground beef and ½ teaspoon salt and cook, stirring frequently, until beef begins to brown,
about 5 minutes. Spoon off fat if necessary. Stir in tomatoes with their
puree, raisins, and olives, breaking up tomatoes with side of spoon, and
cook until sauce thickens slightly, about 5 minutes longer.

3. When pasta has cooked to desired doneness, remove 1 cup pasta
cooking water. Drain pasta and return to saucepot. Add ground-beef
mixture and reserved pasta cooking water; toss well. Add salt to taste.
Garnish with parsley to serve.

Each serving: About 452 calories ▪ 22 g protein ▪ 67 g carbohydrate ▪ 9 g
fiber ▪ 12 g total fat (3 g saturated) ▪ 37 mg cholesterol ▪ 175 mg sodium
(if using reduced-sodium tomatoes).

▶ Penne Rigate for One

If you're serving just yourself, here's a quick, one-portion version: In
boiling water cook *¾ cup dry penne* (preferably whole-wheat) according

to package directions. Meanwhile, in a medium non-stick saucepan, heat *½ teaspoon olive oil*. Add *2 ounces 90% lean round beef* and cook, stirring frequently, 5 minutes. Add *½ cup marinara sauce, 1 tablespoon raisins* and *1 tablespoon chopped olives*.

Each serving: About 441 calories ▪ 21 g protein ▪ 60 g carbohydrate ▪ 8 g fiber ▪ 14 g total fat (3 g saturated) ▪ 37 mg cholesterol ▪ 745 mg sodium.

WEDNESDAY

Breakfast

▶ **Cinnamon-Apple Peanut Butter Toast**

Spread *1 slice whole-wheat toast* with *1 tablespoon peanut or almond butter* and top with slices from *1 small apple* (or half a large apple). Drizzle with *2 teaspoons honey* and sprinkle with *cinnamon*.

Serve with 1 cup fat-free milk and the remainder of the apple.

Snack

⅓ cup grapes (about 11 grapes)

Lunch

Penne Rigate with Sweet-and-Spicy Picadillo Sauce (left over from last night)

Dinner

▶ **Greek Lentil Soup**

Heat *1½ cups canned lentil soup* and *2 cups fresh spinach* (for convenience, use a bag of prewashed spinach). Garnish with *¼ cup crumbled feta cheese*.

Serve with 1 small (4-inch) whole-wheat pita or 1 slice whole-wheat toast.

THURSDAY

Breakfast

Cereal, fruit, and nuts: 190 calories of high-fiber cereal with ½ cup blueberries, 2 tablespoons pecans, and 1 cup fat-free milk.

SuperTip ➤ Slim Down with Fiber

Switching from a low-fiber diet to a high-fiber diet is like taking a weight-loss pill. Studies show that on two diets of the *same number of calories*—one diet high in fiber and one low—people lose more weight on the high-fiber plan. And, looking at it from the flip side, women who eat the most white flour and other refined grains tend to be fatter than women who eat the least, according to Harvard University's long-running study tracking thousands of women and their eating habits. How does fiber work its weight-loss magic? In a number of clever ways:

▶ It's filling. Most obviously, it swells a little in the stomach, suppressing appetite. So 100 calories of Kellogg's All Bran (18 g fiber) would make you feel a lot fuller than 100 calories of corn flakes.

▶ It's low cal. Pure fiber itself has virtually no calories, because the body can't break it down, it just runs right through your digestive system. Cup for cup, or bowl for bowl, or however you want to measure it, high-fiber foods are usually lower in calories than low-fiber foods. For example a cup of apple juice has 0 g fiber and 117 calories; a cup of sliced apple (with skin) has 74 calories and 3.4 g fiber.

▶ It triggers slimming hormonal signals in both men and women. Many high-fiber foods, such as oatmeal, keep blood sugar moderate, which keeps levels of the hormone insulin low. Low insulin is linked to lower body fat (and lower risk of diabetes). Also, bacteria in the gut feed on fiber, raising levels of hormones that send "I'm full!" messages to the brain.

▶ It removes some fat. Some types of fiber, particularly those in fruits and vegetables, trap a little fat from the meal, sweeping it out before the body absorbs it.

Foods high in fiber include fruit, vegetables, beans (legumes), wheat bran, oat bran, corn bran, breads, cereals, pasta, and other starchy foods made with whole grains (such as oats, whole wheat, and whole rye). For more on whole grains see "How to Spot the Whole Grain in the Ingredients List" on page 164.

Lunch
▶ Turkey and Swiss Sandwich

Stuff *2 slices whole-wheat bread* (or a whole-wheat tortilla) with *2 ounces (about 2 slices) turkey breast* and *1½ ounces (1½ slices) reduced-fat Cheddar or 2% cheese singles.* Spread with *2 teaspoons reduced-fat mayo, mustard to taste,* and *lettuce* and *tomato.*

Have a side salad (i.e., 2 cups mixed greens) with 1 tablespoon light dressing.

Dinner

Microwavable meal: As previously noted, look for meals with 400 to 420 calories and at least 5 g fiber and no more than 3 g saturated fat.

Snack

Frozen fruit juice bar, no more than 70 calories

FRIDAY
Breakfast
▶ Smoothie

In a blender, combine *¾ cup plain low-fat yogurt, ½ cup fat-free milk, 1 cup fresh or frozen strawberries, 1 ripe banana,* and *1 teaspoon honey.* If using fresh strawberries, add *2 ice cubes.* Blend until smooth. Pour the mixture into a tall glass or take it with you in a thermos.

Serve with 2 tablespoons nuts.

Lunch
▶ Bean Burrito

Fill a warm *whole-wheat tortilla* (no more than 120 calories) with *½ cup canned refried beans* (about 120 calories per ½ cup, such as Amy's brand), *¼ avocado, 2 to 3 tablespoons salsa,* and *½ slice reduced-fat cheese,* torn into smaller pieces. Roll and serve.

If you're eating out: At Taco Bell, have the regular Bean Burrito; at Baja Fresh, have three fourths of the Vegetarian Bare Burrito (leave one fourth on your plate).

Dinner

Pizza, salad, and beer! 2 slices medium (12-inch) vegetarian pizza (not thick crust) or 2½ slices medium thin-crust vegetarian pizza (e.g., Domino's 12-inch Crunchy Thin-Crust Green Pepper, Onion & Mushroom) or 380 calories of any frozen vegetarian pizza.

Serve with a 12-ounce light beer or 8-ounce regular soft drink or juice and a salad (2 cups mixed greens dressed with 1 teaspoon olive oil and vinegar or lemon juice to taste).

SATURDAY

Breakfast

▶ Egg Burrito

In a nonstick skillet, make scrambled eggs with *2 eggs* and about *2 tablespoons salsa*. Roll into a warmed, *8-inch whole-wheat tortilla* (100 to 120 calories, e.g., Cedar Lane brand). Or, substitute Amy's Breakfast Burrito.

Serve with café au lait (1 cup brewed coffee, regular or decaf, mixed with 1 cup fat-free hot milk) and a slice of cantaloupe (¼ of a medium melon) or another seasonal fruit of your choice.

Lunch

▶ Veggie Cheeseburger

Prepare a *110- to 120-calorie soy-based vegetable burger* according to package directions. (Boca All-American Flame-Grilled or Gardenburger Flame-Grilled are soy-based, meaning that soy is the first or second ingredient.) Melt *1 ounce (1 slice) reduced-fat cheese*, such as Cabot 50% Cheddar or Kraft 2% Singles, on patty during last stages of cooking. Place on a *whole-wheat bun* (about 115 calories) spread with *mustard* and *ketchup* to taste, along with slices of *tomato, onion,* and *lettuce*.

Serve with ½ cup baby carrots.

Snack

1 cup fat-free milk

Dinner
▶ Parsley Pesto Salmon
Prep: 10 minutes ■ Cook: 12 minutes ■ Makes 4 servings

1 cup chopped fresh parsley
¼ cup olive oil
2 tablespoons lemon juice
½ teaspoon salt
¼ teaspoon pepper
4 salmon steaks, about ¾ inch thick (about 4 ounces each)

1. Preheat oven to 400°F. In blender or in food processor with knife blade attached, puree parsley, oil, lemon juice, salt, and pepper until smooth.

2. Coat salmon steaks with parsley mixture. In ovenproof 10-inch skillet over high heat, cook until salmon is lightly browned on both sides, about 2 minutes.

3. Place skillet in oven. Bake salmon until just opaque throughout, about 10 minutes.

Each serving: About 334 calories ■ 23 g protein ■ 2 g carbohydrate ■ 1 g fiber ■ 21 g total fat (4 g saturated) ■ 67 mg cholesterol ■ 366 mg sodium.

Or, if you're really pressed for time, simply broil or grill 4 ounces of salmon seasoned with salt and pepper to taste and sprinkle with chopped parsley, if desired.

▶ Watercress Salad
In salad bowl, mix together *2 teaspoons olive oil, a dash of vinegar or fresh lemon juice to taste,* and *salt and pepper to taste.* Add a *dash of garlic powder or ⅛ teaspoon finely chopped garlic,* if desired. Add *1 cup watercress* mixed with *2 cups milder-tasting greens* such as romaine or butterhead lettuce and toss until greens are evenly coated.

If you're eating out: Order 3 ounces grilled salmon (deck of cards size) or 6 ounces of a white grilled fish. Request no butter sauce on the fish. Add an all-vegetable salad and dress it yourself, lightly.

SUNDAY

Breakfast

Cereal, fruit, and nuts: 190 calories of high-fiber cereal with ½ cup blueberries, 2 tablespoons pecans, and 1 cup fat-free milk.

Lunch

▶ Peanut Butter and Apple Sandwich

Spread *2 slices whole-wheat bread* with a total of *2 tablespoons peanut butter* (or almond butter). Layer with slices from *1 small apple.*

Serve with 1 cup fat-free milk and 1 cup crudités (e.g., broccoli, cauliflower, red pepper, etc.) dipped in light ranch dressing.

Dinner

▶ Curried Chicken and Mango Salad

Precooked chicken from the deli or supermarket makes our salad a cinch. The recipe can easily be doubled if you need to feed a crowd.
Prep: 20 minutes ■ Makes 4 servings

1 store-bought rotisserie chicken (about 2 pounds)
1/4 cup plain low-fat yogurt
1/4 cup reduced-fat mayonnaise
2 tablespoons mango chutney, chopped
1 tablespoon fresh lime juice
1 teaspoon curry powder
1 ripe large mango, peeled and diced
1 medium stalk celery, diced
1 medium Granny Smith apple, cored and diced
1/2 cup loosely packed fresh cilantro leaves, chopped
1 head lettuce, separated and rinsed
cilantro leaves for garnish

1. Remove skin from chicken; discard. With fingers, pull chicken meat into 1-inch pieces. (You should have about 3 cups or about ¾ pound meat.)

2. In large bowl, mix yogurt, mayonnaise, chutney, lime juice, and curry powder until combined. Stir in chicken, mango, celery, apple, and

Good Fats, Bad Fats

Remember when it seemed as though half the products in the supermarket were "low-fat" or "fat-free"—even raspberry Danishes! As we've learned more about fats, it's turned out that not all fat, but *certain* fats, are linked to heart disease and other ills. Throughout this book, you'll read more about "good" and "bad" fats. Here's a little introduction:

Good Fats. These fats—monounsaturated and polyunsaturated—do not raise cholesterol. Polyunsaturated fat is divided into two types: omega-6 and omega-3 (named after their chemical structures). The omega-6 type is fine in moderation, but it's not as all-around healthful as monounsaturated fat, so don't make the omega-6–rich oils your staples. Omega-3s are famous for helping reduce the risk of heart disease, depression, and arthritis symptoms. Keep in mind that good fats are just as high in calories as bad fats, so your goal is to replace saturated and trans fats with these healthy fats and add them to your regular diet!

▶ Monounsaturated fat is plentiful in

☐ almonds ☐ cashews
☐ avocados ☐ olive oil
☐ canola oil ☐ peanuts

Canola and olive oil should be your staples.

▶ Polyunsaturated fat:

Omega-6s:

☐ corn oil ☐ soybean oil
☐ safflower oil ☐ sunflower oil

(unless any of these oils' nutrition labels state that they are "high oleic." This means they are higher in monounsaturated and lower in polyunsaturated fat).

Omega-3s: Two types—EPA and DHA—come from fish oils. Most white fish is low in oil of any type, but bluefish, herring, salmon, sardines, and trout are rich sources of omega-3s. ALA is a plant source of omega-3 found in

☐ canola oil ☐ flaxseeds
☐ edamame (young green soybeans) ☐ walnuts
☐ flaxseed oil ☐ wheat germ

Bad Fats. These are saturated and trans fats, which raise blood cholesterol and are linked to heart disease, inflammation, and, perhaps, cancer. Trans fat is even worse than saturated fat because it not only raises levels of LDL ("bad" cholesterol) but lowers levels of HDL ("good" cholesterol").

▶ Saturated fat is plentiful in

☐ butter
☐ chicken skin
☐ coconut oil
☐ cottonseed oil
☐ palm oil
☐ fatty cuts of meat

While you can't eliminate saturated fat from your diet—little bits of it are also found in oils rich in healthy fats, such as olive oil—you *can* cut back. *The Supermarket Diet* plans are low in saturated fat.

▶ Most trans fat is man-made, created by a process called hydrogenation which converts oils ino firmer fats, such as margarine and shortening. Cookies, piecrusts, snack foods, crackers, breading, and other products with "partially hydrogenated" oils or "shortening" on the label are sources of trans fat. Since the government is now requiring manufacturers to list trans fat on the label, some companies are removing sources of this fat from their products. Very few foods in *The Supermarket Diet* contain trans fat.

Super Tip: ➤ How to Remember Which Fats Are Bad for You

Simple! Just think of this little rhyme: Bad Fats are Trans Sats.

cilantro until well coated. Serve salad on bed of lettuce leaves. Garnish with cilantro leaves.

Each serving: About 323 calories ■ 33 g protein ■ 23 g carbohydrate ■ 3 g fiber ■ 12 g total fat (3 g saturated) ■ 98 mg cholesterol ■ 213 mg sodium.

2 Week Two ➤ Boot Camp Recipes

MONDAY

Breakfast
▶ **Apple Oatmeal with Brown Sugar**

Cook *½ cup plain oatmeal* with *½ cup fat-free milk, ⅓ cup water,* and *1 small apple,* cored and chopped. Serve topped with *cinnamon, 2 teaspoons brown sugar, and 2 tablespoons chopped almonds or walnuts.*

Serve ½ cup fat-free milk with the oatmeal or in a glass.

Lunch
Curried Chicken and Mango Salad (left over from last night's dinner): Have one serving (one fourth of the entire recipe).

Snack
½ cup plain yogurt mixed with 1 teaspoon honey and 5 pecan halves.

Dinner
▶ **Shrimp and Pineapple Stir-Fry**

Have one fourth of the recipe and save another fourth for tomorrow.
Prep: 5 minutes ■ Cook: 12 minutes ■ Makes 4 servings

1 cup quick-cooking brown rice
2 teaspoons canola oil
1 bag (16 ounces) fresh mixed cut vegetables (broccoli, carrot, snap pea, and celery blend)
⅓ cup bottled stir-fry sauce
2 teaspoons cornstarch
1 pound frozen raw shelled and deveined large shrimp
1 can (8 ounces) pineapple chunks in juice

1. Prepare rice as label directs.

2. Meanwhile, in nonstick 12-inch skillet, heat oil over medium-high heat until hot. Add vegetables and cook, stirring constantly, until evenly coated with oil. Cover skillet and cook, stirring occasionally, until vegetables are tender-crisp, 3 to 4 minutes longer.

3. In 1-cup liquid measure, combine stir-fry sauce and cornstarch; stir until blended. Add shrimp, pineapple with its juice, and stir-fry-sauce mixture to vegetables in skillet; cook, stirring occasionally, just until shrimp turn opaque throughout, 4 to 5 minutes.

4. To serve, spoon rice onto 4 dinner plates; top with shrimp mixture.
Each serving: About 349 calories ▪ 27 g protein ▪ 44 g carbohydrate ▪ 4 g fiber ▪ 6 g total fat (1 g saturated) ▪ 172 mg cholesterol ▪ 530 mg sodium.

TUESDAY

Breakfast

❯ Nut Butter and Toast

Spread *2 slices whole-wheat bread* with a total of *4 teaspoons peanut or almond butter* and *4 teaspoons jam, jelly, or honey.*

Serve with 1 cup fat-free milk and an orange

Lunch

Shrimp and Pineapple Stir-Fry (left over from last night's dinner): Have one serving (one fourth of the recipe).

Dinner

❯ Cuban-Style Black Bean Soup

Top *1½ cups canned black bean soup* with *1 to 2 tablespoons plain low-fat yogurt, 1 chopped scallion,* and *2 teaspoons chopped cilantro,* if desired.

Serve the soup with 1 slice bread of any type. For dessert, have 1 cup strawberries or ½ cup blueberries topped with ⅓ cup plain low-fat yogurt sweetened with 1 teaspoon honey.

WEDNESDAY

Breakfast

Cereal, fruit, and nuts: 190 calories of high-fiber cereal with ½ cup blueberries, raspberries, or blackberries, 2 tablespoons chopped pecans, and 1 cup fat-free milk.

Lunch

▶ Pita and Hummus

Stuff a *6-inch whole-wheat pita* with *⅓ cup hummus* and *1 slice (1 ounce) reduced-fat Swiss or Cheddar*. Add *tomato slices*.

Serve with the remainder of the tomato, sliced, on top of mixed greens dressed with 1 tablespoon light dressing.

Buy store-bought hummus, or, if you'd like, make your own.

▶ Hummus

Prep: 15 minutes plus chilling. ■ Makes 2 cups

4 cloves garlic, peeled
1 large lemon
1 can (15 to 19 ounces) garbanzo beans, rinsed and drained
2¹/₂ tablespoons tahini (sesame seed paste)
1 tablespoon olive oil
2 tablespoons water
¹/₄ teaspoon salt
¹/₈ teaspoon ground red pepper (cayenne), optional
¹/₂ teaspoon paprika
2 tablespoons chopped fresh parsley or cilantro (optional)

1. In 1-quart saucepan, heat *2 cups water* to boiling over high heat. Add garlic and cook 3 minutes; drain.

2. From lemon, grate 1 teaspoon peel and squeeze 3 tablespoons juice. In food processor with knife blade attached, combine beans, tahini, garlic, lemon peel and juice, oil, water, salt, and ground red pepper; puree until smooth. Transfer to a platter, cover, and refrigerate up to 4 hours.

3. To serve, sprinkle with paprika and parsley or cilantro, if using.

Each serving (about ⅓ cup): About 157 calories ■ 5 g protein ■ 21 g carbohydrate ■ 4 g fiber ■ 6 g total fat (1 g saturated) ■ 0 mg cholesterol ■ 243 mg sodium.

Dinner

▶ Spaghetti with Meat Sauce

In a heavy skillet with no oil, gently cook *4 ounces crumbled 95% lean ground beef* until cooked through. Add *⅓ cup marinara sauce* and heat through. Mix sauce with *1 cup cooked whole-wheat spaghetti, penne, or other pasta* of your choice.

Serve with 1 cup steamed broccoli seasoned with fresh lemon juice and a little garlic powder, if desired.

THURSDAY

Breakfast

Yogurt, fruit, and nuts: 1 cup (8 ounces) plain low-fat yogurt with 2 teaspoons honey or maple syrup, 3 tablespoons chopped nuts of your choice, and 1 small cored and chopped apple.

Lunch

▶ Greek Salad

You can make this yourself the night before and add the dressing at work, or get it from a restaurant. If the restaurant version has more cheese or olives, leave the extra on the plate. Be sure to request dressing on the side.

Combine *2 cups greens* (mixed greens, Romaine, etc.), *½ cup cucumbers and/or tomatoes, 5 olives, a few onion slices,* and *⅓ cup crumbled feta cheese.* Toss with *1 tablespoon Greek dressing* (2 teaspoons olive oil, ½ teaspoon vinegar, ¼ teaspoon dried oregano, and a dash garlic powder or ¼ teaspoon crushed garlic).

Serve with a 6-inch whole-wheat pita.

Dinner

Rotisserie chicken, corn-on-the-cob, and greens: 1 rotisserie chicken breast (skin removed), microwaved or boiled 5-inch ear of corn (husk and silk removed) and Sautéed Greens.

▶ Sautéed Greens

Wash a *bunch of mustard greens or red or Swiss chard,* remove the tough stems, and chop coarsely. In a heavy skillet, heat *1 tablespoon olive oil* until hot. Add *1 large clove garlic,* cut in half. Add the greens (with the water that clings to the leaves) and sauté over medium heat, stirring occasionally, until thoroughly wilted. Add *salt and pepper to taste* and a sprinkling of *hot pepper flakes,* if desired. Have a third of the greens; reserve at least one third for tomorrow's dinner.

Breakfast
▶ Banana Oatmeal with Brown Sugar
Cook *½ cup plain oats* with *½ cup fat-free milk, ⅓ cup water*, and a *banana*, chopped. Serve topped with *cinnamon, 2 teaspoons brown sugar, 2 tablespoons almonds or walnuts.*

    Serve ½ cup fat-free milk with the oatmeal or in a glass.

Lunch
▶ Roast Beef Sandwich
Spread *2 slices whole-wheat bread* with *2 teaspoons reduced-calorie mayo* and, if desired, *1 tablespoon horseradish or mustard.* Fill the sandwich with *3 ounces lean roast beef* (e.g., Healthy Choice or Boar's Head brand) and *slices of lettuce and tomato.* Have the remainder of the tomato, sliced, sprinkled with a little salt.

Snack
6 ounces flavored light yogurt (about 90 calories)

Dinner
▶ Middle Eastern Mezze
Arrange on a plate: *⅓ cup hummus, ¼ cup crumbled feta, 3 to 4 olives,* and *1 serving of last night's greens* sprinkled with *a little fresh lemon juice.* Drizzle *1 teaspoon olive oil* over the food and scoop it up with *1 (6-inch) whole-wheat pita.*

SATURDAY
Breakfast
▶ Smoothie
In a blender, combine *¾ cup plain low-fat yogurt, ½ cup fat-free milk, 1 cup fresh or frozen strawberries, 1 ripe banana,* and *1 teaspoon honey.* If using fresh strawberries, add *2 ice cubes.* Blend until smooth. Pour the mixture into a tall glass.

    Serve with 2 tablespoons nuts.

Lunch
▶ Chicken Salad with Grapes
Combine *⅔ cup cooked skinless chicken breast* (from a rotisserie chicken or buy precooked white meat chicken slices) with *1 tablespoon reduced-fat*

mayo and *1 tablespoon plain low-fat yogurt.* Add *⅓ cup seedless grapes,* sliced in half, and *2 tablespoons almonds* or any other nuts of your choice. Optional: If available, add *1 or 2 tablespoons chopped celery* and *2 teaspoons chopped fresh dill.* Serve over a bed of *lettuce leaves.*

NOTE: Save ⅓ cup chicken for tomorrow's soup.

Dinner
Asian stir-fry: Order takeout from your local Chinese restaurant or make your own.

No-time version: Order *vegetable/chicken, vegetable/shrimp, or vegetable/tofu stir-fry* and have 1½ cups (avoid anything deep fried—i.e., no "crispy" chicken—and make sure to get "white," not fried, tofu) with *¾ cup steamed rice* (brown rice if they serve it).

Enjoy a 12-ounce light beer or another 100-calorie treat of your choice.

▶ Gingered Pork and Vegetable Stir-Fry
Have 1 serving with ¾ cup rice, preferably brown (Minute rice is fine).
Prep: 15 minutes ▪ Cook: 15 minutes ▪ Makes 4 servings

1 pork tenderloin (12 ounces), thinly sliced
2 tablespoons grated, peeled fresh ginger
1 cup reduced-sodium chicken broth
2 tablespoons teriyaki sauce
2 teaspoons cornstarch
2 teaspoons canola oil
8 ounces snow peas, strings removed
1 medium zucchini (8 ounces), halved lengthwise and thinly
    sliced
3 green onions, cut into 3-inch pieces

1. In medium bowl, toss pork and fresh ginger. In cup, mix broth, teriyaki sauce, and cornstarch; set aside.
2. In nonstick, 12-inch skillet, heat 1 teaspoon oil over medium-high heat until hot. Add snow peas, zucchini, and green onions and cook, stirring frequently (stir-frying), until lightly browned and tender-crisp, about 5 minutes. Transfer to bowl.

3. In same skillet, heat remaining 1 teaspoon oil; add pork mixture and stir-fry until pork just loses its pink color. Transfer pork to bowl with vegetables. Stir cornstarch mixture; add to skillet and heat to boiling. Boil until sauce thickens, about 1 minute. Stir in pork and vegetables; heat through.

Each serving: About 186 calories ▪ 21 g protein ▪ 8 g carbohydrate ▪ 1 g fiber ▪ 8 g total fat (1 g saturated) ▪ 55 mg cholesterol ▪ 430 mg sodium.

SUNDAY

Breakfast

▶ Scrambled Eggs and Toast

Scramble *2 eggs* in *1 teaspoon trans fat–free margarine*. Serve with *1 slice whole-wheat toast* spread with another *teaspoon of the margarine* and *1 cup of fruit* of your choice.

Snack

8 ounces fat-free milk with 1 teaspoon chocolate syrup

Lunch

▶ Curried Butternut Squash Soup with Spinach, Couscous and Chicken

Have 1½ cups. Either open a can or carton, or make your own. Freeze any leftovers in portion sizes. To the soup, add 2 tablespoons couscous (preferably whole-wheat) and 2 handfuls of fresh spinach (use the prewashed, bagged type for convenience) and simmer until the couscous is cooked. Add ⅓ cup cooked chicken (leftover from yesterday) and serve.

Prep: 20 minutes ▪ Cook: 40 minutes ▪ Makes 4 servings (6 cups)

1½ tablespoons trans fat–free margarine
1 large onion (12 ounces), sliced
1½ teaspoons curry powder
1 large butternut squash (1¼ pounds), peeled, seeded, and cut
    into ½-inch chunks
1 can (14½ ounces) reduced-sodium chicken broth
1/4 teaspoon salt

1. In 5-quart Dutch oven or saucepot, melt 1 tablespoon margarine over medium heat. Add onion and cook, stirring occasionally, until golden and tender, 18 to 20 minutes. Add curry and remaining ½ tablespoon margarine and cook, stirring, 1 minute. Add squash, broth, salt, and *1⅛ cups water;* heat to boiling. Reduce heat to low; cover and simmer soup until squash is very tender, about 20 minutes.

2. In blender at low speed, with center part of cover removed to allow steam to escape, blend squash mixture in small batches until very smooth. Pour soup into large bowl after each batch.

3. Return blended soup to Dutch oven; heat through.

Each serving, without spinach, couscous and chicken (about 1½ cups): About 108 calories ▪ 2 g protein ▪ 20 g carbohydrate ▪ 1 g fiber ▪ 3 g total fat (1 g saturated) ▪ 0 mg cholesterol ▪ 195 mg sodium.

Each serving, with 2 tablespoons dry couscous, 2 handfuls spinach, and ⅓ cup cooked skinless chicken breast: About 300 calories ▪ 22 g protein ▪ 44 g carbohydrate ▪ 5g fiber ▪ 6 g total fat (1 g saturated) ▪ 39 mg cholesterol ▪ 371 mg sodium.

Dinner

▶ Trout with Cornmeal Crust and Spicy Corn Relish

Prepare the relish first and then set it aside. Serve the trout and corn with a cup of steamed cauliflower or broccoli, seasoned with a spritz of lemon.

Prep: 25 minutes ▪ Cook: 6 minutes ▪ Makes 4 servings

> 4 brook or rainbow trout fillets (1/4 pound each)
> 3/4 teaspoon salt
> 1/2 teaspoon ground black pepper
> 3 tablespoons yellow cornmeal
> 1 tablespoon all-purpose flour
> 1 teaspoon paprika
> 2 tablespoons canola oil

1. Sprinkle fillets with salt and pepper. On waxed paper, mix cornmeal, flour, and paprika. Dip fillets into cornmeal mixture, turning to coat sides.

2. In 12-inch skillet, heat oil over medium-high heat. Add fish fillets and cook, carefully turning fillets once, until fish is golden brown and opaque throughout, about 6 minutes.

Each serving: About 220 calories ▪ 25 g protein ▪ 7 g carbohydrate ▪ 1 g fiber ▪ 10 g total fat (2 g saturated) ▪ 67 mg cholesterol ▪ 476 mg sodium.

▌ Spicy Corn Relish

Boil *4 ears corn,* husks and silk removed; cut kernels from cobs. In medium bowl, mix corn kernels; *1 large red pepper,* diced; *2 jalepeño chiles,* minced; *2 tablespoons cider vinegar; 1 tablespoon olive or vegetable oil; 1 tablespoon chopped fresh cilantro; ½ teaspoon sugar;* and *¼ teaspoon salt.* Makes about 2½ cups.

4 Keep On Losin' Plan

If you made it through Boot Camp, this next step will be a breeze. You get 300 more calories a day—practically a meal's worth—and loads of flexibility. Keep up the exercise prescription in chapter 5, "Burn the Fat," and you should be losing about a pound a week, maybe more. You can stay on this nutritionally balanced plan for months, even a year.

Men: This chapter's 1,500-calorie plan is your starting point. As explained on page 15, the 1,200-calorie Boot Camp is too low for your greater metabolic needs. Follow this plan for two weeks, then move on to the 1,800-calorie Stay Slim Maintenance plan, chapter 8.

Design Your Day

Feel like eggs for breakfast? Go ahead! Sick of chicken? Have fish tonight instead. With this incredibly flexible program, you get to pick your breakfasts, lunches, dinners, and snacks. All the math has been done for you: All the breakfasts work out to about 375 calories, the lunches are about 400 calories, the dinners 500 calories, plus you get a daily snack. All you've got to do is pick any breakfast, lunch, dinner, and snack from the lists provided. Every meal in any particular category (i.e. breakfast) has a similarly balanced nutrition profile. So, you can't help but design a healthy day. With 400,000 possible combinations, it'll be a long time before you get tired of this plan!

In the "Be Your Own Nutritionist" section on page 130, you'll learn how to use food exchanges to create any meal you desire. So if a favorite meal isn't on the lists, you've got all the tools to turn it into a Keep On Losin' meal.

One of the great features of this plan is that you get to pick a tasty snack every day. Kicking back with a light beer or savoring a creamy chocolate truffle or polishing off a large fruit salad (yes, there are people who actually *prefer* fruit over candy!) does wonders for your morale while you're trying to lose weight. You can relax knowing that you can keep your favorite foods in your life. You do have to watch the portions though, and that's what the snack lists control for you. Every day, you've got 125 calories to play with to bring this weight loss plan up to 1,500 calories a day. Ideally, you should pick a fruit snack at least three days in any week, and have the sweets or other snacky foods on this list the rest of the week. But if having the sweets and snacks is what keeps you on track, then it's OK to choose the fruit snacks less often. The rest of the plan is high enough in fruits and vegetables to keep you healthy.

While you can choose any of the meals on the lists, there are some combos that inject an extra weight-loss (and health) advantage. "Get the Max from Your Meals" (opposite) will guide you to the best ways of approaching this plan. For instance, studies consistently show that people lose more weight on higher-fiber diets than on lower-fiber diets of the same calorie count. Then there are all the health benefits of fiber: lowering the risk of diabetes, heart disease, and certain types of cancer. Most Keep On Losin' meals are fiber-rich, some exceptionally so. But there are still a few comforting favorites—e.g., toast and eggs, and "meat and potatoes"–type dishes—that don't happen to be great sources of fiber. Just balance those with the higher-fiber dishes. (A meal with 8 g fiber or more is considered high fiber.) It's also a good idea to have some vegetarian meals, especially bean-based meals. Plant protein is linked to a reduced risk of cancer and other age-related diseases. Finally, aim for at least two fish meals a week, as the American Heart Association recommends.

Keep On Movin'

Just because you've graduated from two weeks in Boot Camp doesn't mean you can stop exercising. *Au contraire!* Now that you're eating more calories, you must keep it up; you may already be adding more minutes to your exercise routine. As you plan your meals in this chapter, keep up the good work with your aerobics, strength training, and stretching routines detailed in chapter 5.

You should lose between ½ and 1 pound a week on Keep On Losin' (along with exercising). If you're not losing weight, ask yourself: Are you truly following the program? Keep yourself honest by filling out a food diary for at least five days and make sure extra calories aren't making

Get the Max from Your Meals

To make sure you get enough fiber—a proven weight-loss tool—and get the healthy benefits of the occasional vegetarian or fish meal, follow these guidelines.

▶ **Get enough fiber.** Choose meals and snacks that add up to 25 g of fiber or more a day (30 g or more for men). For instance, if you had the Fruit-Topped Waffles breakfast (9 g fiber), a Vegetable Burger with Avocado Salsa (13 g fiber), and Orange-Glazed Steak (6 g fiber) for dinner, you've racked up 28 g of fiber.

▶ **Eat some vegetarian meals.** Try to have one vegetarian meal, in addition to breakfast, daily or nearly every day. Vegetarian meals can include dairy and eggs. This is not a "must," but it's a good habit to get into for long-term health benefits. In the example above, the Fruit-Topped Waffle and the Vegetable Burger with Avocado Salsa were both vegetarian. A great lineup: the Carrot Bran Muffin breakfast (vegetarian), the Chicken Salad Sandwich lunch (not vegetarian), and the Almost Instant Rice Salad dinner (vegetarian).

▶ **Have fish twice a week.** The American Heart Association recommends eating fish twice a week to reduce the risk of heart disease. Fresh, frozen, smoked, or canned, it all counts as fish. A nice lineup: the Cereal and Fruit breakfast, the Smoked Salmon Sandwich for lunch, and the Tuscan White Bean Bruschetta for dinner.

Tweaking the Plan: Do's and Don'ts

Here's what you can—and can't—get away with on the Keep On Losin' plan. You're welcome to tweak meals as long as you don't fiddle much with the calorie counts. Some guidelines:

▶ **Shortening prep time.** The meals on this plan don't take much time or cooking skill. Most meals take just 5 to 25 minutes to prepare. If you don't have the time or inclination to make these exact recipes, no problem; take shortcuts. For instance, if you don't want to make your own skinless chicken breasts, use pre-cooked chicken pieces.

▶ **Subbing ingredients.** It's perfectly OK to use romaine lettuce instead of mixed greens, chopped carrots for celery, flounder for halibut, margarine for oil, or similar swaps. But if you substitute an extra tablespoon of low-fat mayo for yogurt, you're adding 30 calories to the meal. Your rule of thumb: Substitute like foods for like foods. Swap lean protein (chicken) for lean protein (fish, scallops, lean meat, etc.); a fat for another fat (mayo for margarine); a starch for a starch (one slice of bread for $1/2$ cup rice); a fruit for a fruit; almonds for pecans; etc. The "Size Up Your Meal" lists on page 131 will help you figure out which foods are in the same group. While it's OK to make these substitutions occasionally, if you're tweaking this plan a lot, best buy a calorie-counter book or check an online website to make sure you're making equivalent calorie swaps. The U.S. Department of Agriculture's nutrient database website offers nutritional analysis of foods for free (www.nal.usda.gov/fnic/foodcomp/search/). NOTE: The bread in this plan should be 65 to 75 calories per slice, no more—so read labels carefully to determine equivalent portion sizes.

▶ **Switching lunch for dinner (and vice versa).** It's fine to do this, just don't have two of the same meal on the same day. If you have two dinners on the same day, you'll bust your calorie limit. If you have two lunches, you won't get quite enough calories (and may go hungry). Also, dinners tend to have more vegetables, so with two lunches, you may be skimping on this important food group.

▶ **Raising calories.** For some of you, a daily intake of 1,500 calories just isn't enough. Signs that you're not getting enough calories: You're hungry when you shouldn't be (one or two hours after eating); you're losing weight too quickly (more than 2 pounds a week for weeks on end might be too quickly); you don't have the energy to complete your workouts. Try having your calcium break a half hour to an hour before working out or about an hour before your next meal. If this still doesn't ward off hunger, then you may need more calories. Try adding 100 calories at a time to the plan (see page 47 for lists of foods with 100 calories).

▶ **Lowering calories.** In most research studies—and with my clients—1,500 daily calories induce weight loss. In fact, female clients who came to see me eating 1,200 calories or less started losing *more* weight when I switched them to 1,500 calories. (At 1,200 calories, with regular exercise, their body was thinking "starvation" and slowed down their metabolism. It took the extra 300 calories to reassure the body that it's OK to turn metabolism back up.) So, it's OK to take in 1,200 calories for a week or two (1,500 calories for men), but then you need to switch to 1,500 calories (1,800 calories for men) to avoid lowering your metabolism.

their way into your diet. (See page 48 to learn how to fill out the food diary.) If you're truly following this program and still not losing weight after a few weeks, you have a few options. Best strategy: Exercise more. If you find the exercises in chapter 5 fairly easy, then increase their intensity and the amount of time you spend working out. If that doesn't work, then use the 100-calorie lists on page 47 to shave off 200 calories. Or, go back to the Boot Camp meal plans for another few weeks.

OK. Now you know the basics of Keep On Losin'. So get ready, set, eat!

Keep On Losin' Menus

375-CALORIE BREAKFASTS

You'll find the simple recipes and notes on how to prepare your Keep On Losin' meals in the recipe section starting on page 84.

Blender Breakfast No. 1: Strawberry Smoothie   9 g fiber
Blender Breakfast No. 2: Peach Smoothie   7 g fiber
Bran muffin and fruit   9 g fiber
Cereal and fruit   15 g fiber
Convenience-store breakfast   5 g fiber
Deli breakfast   7 g fiber
Eggs and toast   5 g fiber
Fruit-topped waffles   9 g fiber
Hot cereal, fruit, and nuts   7 g fiber
Nut butter and toast   5 g fiber
Yogurt, fruit, and nuts   5 g fiber

400-CALORIE LUNCHES

Hot Meals
Baked Potato Stuffed with Chili   7 g fiber
Cafeteria meal   3 g fiber
Grilled cheese and lentil soup   11 g fiber

Salads
Garbanzo Salad   11 g fiber
Salad-bar Salad   13 g fiber
Spinach Salad with Orange   8 g fiber
Tuna and Cannellini Bean Salad   11 g fiber
Waldorf Salad with turkey   6 g fiber

Sandwiches/Burritos
Chicken Salad Sandwich with broccoli   5 g fiber
Classic Tuna Salad Sandwich with carrots and celery   7 g fiber
Health Club Sandwich   11 g fiber
Hummus Sandwich   13 g fiber

Peanut Butter and Jelly Sandwich   7 g fiber
Smoked Salmon Sandwich with salad   6 g fiber
Turkey and Swiss Sandwich with salad   8 g fiber
Vegetarian Black Bean Burrito with crudités   15 g fiber
Vegetarian Burger with salad   13 g fiber

Soups
Entire-Meal Tomato Soup   12 g fiber
Italian White Bean and Spinach Soup with crackers   16 g fiber
Black bean soup with cheese and crackers   17 g fiber

500-CALORIE DINNERS
Beef and Pork
Burger and "fries"   5 g fiber
Filet Mignon with Tomatoes and Roquefort   6 g fiber
Orange-Glazed Steak with Pear and Blue Cheese Salad, and sweet potato
    6 g fiber
Pork Steak with Plum Glaze and Lemon-Parsley Rice with zucchini
    5 g fiber

Chicken
Chicken Caesar Salad with sweet potato   9 g fiber
Chicken with couscous and spinach   11 g fiber
Rotisserie chicken with sweet potato and Roasted Cauliflower   7 g fiber
Texas Chicken Burger with broccoli   13 g fiber

Fish and Shellfish
Grilled Halibut with grilled vegetables and beer   8 g fiber
Honey-Lime Salmon with salad and garlic bread   4 g fiber
Scallops with Watercress, with bulgur wheat   5 g fiber
Snapper Livornese with Lemon-Parsley Rice and broccoli   7 g fiber
Tuscan Tuna Salad Pita with salad   8 g fiber

Pasta and Rice
Pad Thai with spinach   4 g fiber
Penne with Salmon and Asparagus   9 g fiber
Whole-wheat pasta with Marinara Sauce with salad   13 g fiber

Vegetarian

Almost-Instant Rice Salad   14 g fiber

Avocado and Black Bean Salad   27 g fiber

Tuscan White Bean Bruschetta with salad   8 g fiber

Vegetable Pizza with salad   12 g fiber

CALCIUM BREAK

One hundred calories each. Have one a day so that you can keep up your essential calcium intake.

Cheese and crackers

Chocolate Milk

Cool Cucumber Soup

Flavored Steamer

Hot Chocolate

Flavored Yogurt

Skim milk

Skim-milk latte

Soy or rice milk, calcium-enriched

SNACKS AND ALCOHOL

Have just one from one category, per day. For instance, have one fruit snack OR one sweet snack OR one salty snack OR one drink. But don't have more than one (i.e., a fruit snack *and* a salty snack).

Fruit Snacks (125 calories each)

See recipe list on page 124 for portions.

Apple and cheddar

Berries and honey yogurt

Broiled Brown Sugar Banana

Dried fruit and nuts

Fruit

Fresh fruit salad

Herb-Poached Peach

Juice

Mini smoothies

Peanut butter–stuffed dates

Sweet Snacks (125 calories each)
See recipe list on page 127 for portions.
Angel food cake

Chocolate

Chocolate-covered peanuts

Cookies

Flan or pudding

Frozen fruit juice bar

Hard candy

Ice cream (light) or frozen yogurt with chocolate syrup

Jelly beans

Malted milk balls

Mini donuts

Salty Snacks (125 calories each)
See recipe list on page 128 for portions.
Chips and dip

Popcorn

Potato chips

Pretzels

Salted nuts

Spinach snacks

Venison or turkey jerky

Whole-wheat crackers with cream cheese and smoked salmon

Alcohol (125 calories each)
See recipe list on page 129 for portions.
Beer, regular or light

Bloody Mary

Daiquiri

Gin and Tonic

Hard liquor

Margarita

Martini

Wine, red or white

Wine cooler

Keep On Losin' Recipes

Again, you'll find that some of the recipes, particularly main dishes for dinner, yield more than one portion. *The Supermarket Diet* assumes that you may be cooking for more than one person. Remember—for family members who are not on the diet, you can simply increase the size of their portions. If you find you have leftovers, simply freeze them for later use.

375-Calorie Breakfasts

A few things to bear in mind about breakfast: You are free to add coffee or tea to any of the breakfasts. If you use sugar, remember, you're adding an extra 16 calories per teaspoon. Soy milk may be substituted for fat-free milk. Check the soy milk label to be sure that it's enriched with calcium (at least 30% of the DV for calcium) and no more than 100 calories per cup. And if you can't use an entire cup of milk in the cereal or oatmeal, drink the rest in a glass or add it to your coffee.

▶ **Blender Breakfast No. 1: Strawberry Smoothie** (9 g fiber)
Prep: 5 minutes plus freezing ▪ Makes 1 serving (2 cups)

> 1 cup calcium-enriched soy milk (about 100 calories and at
>   least 25% of the DV for calcium per cup)
> 1 frozen banana, sliced
> 1 cup strawberries, hulled
> 2 tablespoons wheat germ
> 1 tablespoon honey

In a blender, combine soy milk, banana, strawberries, wheat germ, and honey; blend until mixture is smooth and frothy. Pour into a tall glass.
Each smoothie: About 370 calories ▪ 13 g protein ▪ 70 g carbohydrate ▪ 9 g fiber ▪ 7 g total fat (1 g saturated) ▪ 0 mg cholesterol ▪ 124 sodium.

▶ Blender Breakfast No. 2: Peach Smoothie (7 g fiber)

Prep: 5 minutes ■ Makes 1 serving (2 cups)

½ cup fat-free milk
½ cup low-fat plain yogurt
1 banana, sliced
1 large peach, peeled and cut into chunks, or 1 cup strawberries, hulled
2 teaspoons honey
1 ice cube

In a blender, combine milk, yogurt, banana, peach, honey, and ice cube; blend until smooth. Pour into a tall glass. Serve with almonds.
Each smoothie (without the almonds): About 327 calories ■ 13 g protein ■ 67 g carbohydrate ■ 6 g fiber ■ 3 g total fat (2 g saturated) 10 mg cholesterol ■ 152 mg sodium.

▶ Bran muffin and fruit (9 g fiber)

Serve 1 muffin with 1 cup fat-free milk and a mix of 1 cup strawberries and ½ cup sliced banana.

▶ Carrot-Bran Muffins

Prep: 15 minutes plus standing ■ Bake: 30 minutes ■ Makes 12 muffins

1 cup low-fat (1%) milk
¼ cup canola oil
1 large egg, lightly beaten
1½ cups whole-bran cereal (not bran flakes)
1 cup shredded carrots
1¼ cups all-purpose flour
⅓ cup sugar
1 tablespoon baking powder
½ teaspoon salt
¼ teaspoon ground cinnamon
1 cup dark seedless raisins

1. Preheat oven to 400°F. Grease twelve 2½ by 1¼-inch muffin-pan cups.

2. In medium bowl, with fork, beat milk, oil, egg, cereal, and carrots until blended; let stand 10 minutes.

3. Meanwhile, in large bowl, combine flour, sugar, baking powder, salt, and cinnamon. Add cereal mixture to flour mixture; stir just until dry ingredients are moistened (batter will be lumpy). Stir in raisins.

4. Spoon batter into prepared muffin-pan cups. Bake until muffins begin to brown and toothpick inserted in center of muffin comes out clean, about 30 minutes. Immediately remove muffins from pan. Serve warm, or cool on wire rack to serve later.

Each muffin: About 185 calories ▪ 4 g protein ▪ 33 g carbohydrate ▪ 4 g fiber ▪ 6 g total fat (1 g saturated) ▪ 19 mg cholesterol ▪ 259 mg sodium.

Cereal and fruit (15 g fiber)

170 calories high-fiber cereal (check labels: should have at least 10 g fiber per 170 calories, see page 183 for suggested brands), topped with ½ cup blueberries, raspberries, or a small chopped apple or half a banana, sliced, and 2 tablespoon almonds, pecans, or other nuts. Serve with 1 cup fat-free milk

Convenience-store breakfast (5 g fiber)

Grab a banana, an 8-ounce carton of fat-free milk, and a 1 ounce-package of peanuts or other nuts.

Deli breakfast (7 g fiber)

Have half of a large whole-wheat bagel spread with 2 tablespoons of light, reduced-fat (not the grainy, bad-tasting fat-free) cream cheese, a 12-ounce skim (fat-free milk) latte, and 1 cup fruit.

Eggs and toast (7 g fiber)

Scramble 2 eggs in 1 teaspoon trans fat–free margarine. Serve with 1 slice whole-wheat toast, 1 cup strawberries, and 1 cup fat-free milk.

Or poach or boil the 2 eggs and serve them with 1 slice whole-wheat toast spread with trans fat–free margarine, plus berries and milk.

Super Tip ➤ Berry Big Nutrition

The Supermarket Diet takes advantage of recent research that shows the extraordinary health benefits of berries. You'll find berries in many of the breakfasts as well as some snacks. Blueberries got lots of buzz after studies at Tufts University/USDA Research Center on Aging in Boston showed that a blueberry extract–enriched diet improved memory and coordination in aging lab rats. Turns out that blueberry extract actually stimulated the growth of new memory cells in the rats' brains. (The rats consumed the human equivalent of 1 cup of blueberries daily.) Powerful antioxidant compounds called *anthocyanins* are getting the credit for the brain boosting.

Blackberries are rich in another exotic beneficial compound: *epicatechin.* It helps prevent and fight cancer, and also fights inflammation, which may also reduce the risk of heart disease. And blackberries are a great source of fiber, at 4 g per half cup. Raspberries are also loaded with 4 g of fiber per ½ cup. And, raspberries boast both epicatechin and high levels of anthocyanins, although not in the stratospheric levels of blueberries. A half cup of strawberries provides 57 percent of your daily requirement for vitamin C, and they are rich in ellagic acid, another cancer-fighting plant compound.

Elderberries, black currants, and chokeberries, all purple berries, are still scarce in the marketplace, but that may change, as consumers learn about their high antioxidant content. U.S. Department of Agriculture research shows that these fruits, particularly elderberries and chokeberries, may have antioxidant levels 50 percent higher than those of the more commonly eaten berries, such as blueberries and blackberries, so they may help fight heart disease and cancer.

Note: Have this breakfast no more than three times a week, since it's lower in fiber than the others. While most research shows that eggs *don't* raise blood cholesterol—despite being high in cholesterol they are low in saturated fat—if you have high cholesterol, check with your doctor about how many eggs you should have per week. Let the doc know that the rest of this plan is low to moderate in cholesterol and saturated fat.

Fruit-topped waffles (9 g fiber)

Have 2 whole-grain waffles, about 170 calories for two (e.g., Kashi brand), topped with a total of 2 teaspoons trans fat–free margarine, 2 teaspoons maple or pancake syrup, and 1 cup frozen or fresh strawberries or half a banana, sliced. Serve with 1 cup fat-free milk.

Hot cereal, fruit, and nuts (7 g fiber)

Make ⅓ cup plain oatmeal according to package directions. (For creamier oats, stir together the dry oats and ⅓ cup *each* water and fat-free milk. Heat, stirring, until cooked.) Top with 1 small apple, sliced, or half a banana (or cook the fruit along with the oatmeal). Sweeten with 1 teaspoon brown sugar or maple syrup and top with 2 tablespoons nuts of your choice and dash of cinnamon. Have 1 cup fat-free milk with the breakfast (some of it may be used to make the oatmeal).

Nut butter and toast (5 g fiber)

Spread 1½ slices whole-wheat bread or toast with 4 teaspoons (total) of almond or peanut butter and 1 teaspoon honey. Top with half a banana, sliced. Serve with 1 cup fat-free milk.

Yogurt, fruit, and nuts (5 g fiber)

Stir together ¾ cup plain low-fat yogurt, 2 teaspoons honey, 1 sliced peach, ½ cup blueberries (or other fruit of your choice), and 3 tablespoons almonds, pecans, cashews, or other nuts.

Attention Shoppers! ➤ Margarine or Butter?

For years we were told that margarine was better for us than butter because butter's saturated fat and cholesterol were so heart-risky. Then it turned out that trans fat—created when liquid vegetable oils are hardened to create margarine—is even worse for you than saturated fat! So, should you go back to butter? Nope, unless it's only an occasional pat or two. On the Keep On Losin' plan you've got a daily saturated-fat limit of 15 grams; a pat of butter (about 1 teaspoon) has 2.5 g. So, you see why you still have to limit butter.

The healthiest alternative: margarine labeled *0 trans fat* or *trans fat free*. It's usually a little softer than the old stick margarines, but it tastes and acts just the same. See our guide on page 198.

The process that creates trans fat in margarine is called *hydrogenation*. Those "partially hydrogenated" oils you see on labels? They've got trans fat. Manufacturers are starting to eliminate or reduce these unhealthy fats in foods now that they're forced to label trans fat. (See "Good Fats, Bad Fats" on page 64).

400-Calorie Lunches

HOT MEALS

▶ **Baked Potato Stuffed with Chili** (7 g fiber)
Have 1 serving.
Prep: 20 minutes ▪ Bake: 45 minutes (15 minutes in microwave—5 minutes for 1 potato) ▪ Makes 4 servings

4 medium baking potatoes (about 7½ ounces each)
12 ounces 95% lean ground beef
1 small onion, chopped
3 tablespoons chili powder
1 can (14½ ounces) chili-style chunky tomatoes
¾ cup water
1 teaspoon sugar

1. Preheat oven to 450°F. With fork, pierce potatoes. Place potatoes directly on oven rack and bake until fork-tender, about 45 minutes. Or bake in microwave, 15 minutes (or 5 minutes for 1 potato).

2. Meanwhile, prepare chili: Heat nonstick 12-inch skillet over medium high heat. Add beef and onion; cook, stirring, until meat is browned and onion is tender. Stir in chili powder; cook 1 minute. Add tomatoes, water, and sugar; cook 1 minute longer.

3. When potatoes are done, slash tops, press to open slightly, and spoon on topping.

Each stuffed potato: About 378 calories ▪ 26 g protein ▪ 58 g carbohydrate ▪ 7 g fiber ▪ 6 g total fat (2 g saturated) ▪ 53 mg cholesterol ▪ 354 mg sodium.

Cafeteria meal (3 g fiber)

Have meat, poultry, or fish that you can make at home and bring to eat at work, e.g., a chicken leg and thigh, skin removed. Or 1 slice of beef, about the size of the palm of your hand. Or a fillet of white fish, about the size of your entire hand, or a small salmon steak (palm size). The meats should have none—or very little—oil, butter, or other sauce. Round out the meal with 1 cup rice and 1 cup steamed broccoli or other vegetable.

Grilled cheese and lentil soup (11 g fiber)

Top 2 slices whole-wheat bread each with 1 slice (1 or 2 ounces total) reduced-fat Cheddar (e.g., Cabot 50% reduced or any of the 2% singles). Heat open-faced, in toaster oven or oven, until cheese has melted. Top 1 slice with sliced tomatoes and sprinkle with a little chopped fresh

Attention Shoppers! ➤ Get Your Potassium-Rich Produce

You've probably heard about sodium raising blood pressure, and it's true. But you hear less about getting enough potassium, an element that helps *lower* blood pressure. Getting enough potassium helps reduce the effects of sodium on blood pressure, and it may reduce kidney stone risk and help decrease age-related bone loss.

Aim for 4,700 mg potassium daily, through food, not supplements. Fruits and vegetables are the best sources not only because they are high in potassium but also because they contain a form that's more easily absorbed by the body than the potassium in milk, meat, and grains.

Some particularly potassium-rich foods:

▶ bananas, plantains
▶ beans (black, kidney, white, etc.)
▶ cantaloupe and honeydew melons
▶ cooked greens (such as spinach, beet greens)
▶ oranges, orange juice
▶ soybeans, both green (edamame) and mature
▶ sweet potatoes
▶ tomato products (sauce, paste, puree)
▶ white potatoes
▶ winter squash (such as butternut)

basil, if desired. Close sandwich and cut in half. Serve with remaining tomato, sliced, and 1 cup canned lentil soup.

SALADS

▶ **Garbanzo Salad** (11 g fiber)
Have 1 serving.
Prep: 20 minutes ■ Makes 2 servings

2 tablespoons red wine vinegar
2 tablespoons olive oil
1 teaspoon Dijon mustard
¼ teaspoon salt
3 small tomatoes (about 12 ounces), each cut into 8 wedges
½ cup Kalamata olives, pitted and coarsely chopped
1 green onion, thinly sliced
1 can (15 ounces) garbanzo beans, rinsed and drained
2 tablespoons chopped fresh oregano, basil, or parsley

1. Prepare vinaigrette: In medium bowl, with wire whisk or fork, mix vinegar, oil, mustard, and salt.
2. Add tomato wedges, olives, green onion, garbanzo beans, and oregano to vinaigrette in bowl; toss until evenly coated.
Each serving: About 397 calories ▪ 14 g protein ▪ 41 g carbohydrate ▪ 11 g fiber ▪ 21 g total fat (2 g saturated) ▪ 0 mg cholesterol ▪ 861 mg sodium.

▶ Salad-Bar Salad (13 g fiber)
Start with *3 cups mixed greens or romaine* (undressed) and pile on about *¼ cup grated carrots, ½ cup green or red pepper rings, 8 cherry tomatoes, ½ cup garbanzo beans,* and *½ cup plain (undressed) chicken or tuna.* Toss with *1 tablespoon regular dressing* or *2 tablespoons reduced-fat dressing.* Serve with *2 or 3 little crackers* or *2 tablespoons croutons.*

▶ Spinach Salad with Orange (8 g fiber)
Have 1 serving of salad with 1½ slices toast with 1 teaspoon trans fat–free margarine.
Prep: 10 minutes ▪ Makes 2 servings

2 large navel oranges
1 tablespoon extravirgin olive oil
¼ teaspoon salt
⅛ teaspoon ground black pepper
6 cups baby spinach
2 hard-cooked eggs, cut in half

1. From 1 orange, grate ½ teaspoon peel and squeeze 3 tablespoons juice. With knife, cut peel and white pith from remaining whole orange. Slice orange crosswise in half, then cut each half into ¼-inch-thick slices; set aside.

2. In medium bowl, whisk oil, salt, pepper, and orange peel and juice. Add spinach; toss to coat.

3. To serve, divide spinach mixture between two salad plates; top with orange and egg halves.

Each serving: About 299 calories ▪ 17 g protein ▪ 21 g carbohydrate ▪ 6 g fiber ▪ 18 g total fat (4 g saturated) ▪ 424 mg cholesterol ▪ 487 mg sodium.

▶ **Tuna and Cannellini Bean Salad** (11 g fiber)
Have 1 serving.
Prep: 12 minutes ▪ Makes 2 servings

1 lemon
1½ cups canned white kidney beans (cannellini), rinsed and
    drained
½ cup coarsely chopped carrots
½ cup chopped tomato (or, if not in season, use red pepper)
1 tablespoon olive oil
2 tablespoons chopped fresh parsley or other herb of your
    choice
⅛ teaspoon coarsely ground pepper
1 can (6 ounces) light tuna, drained

1. From lemon, finely grate ½ teaspoon peel and squeeze 1 tablespoon juice.

2. In medium serving bowl, combine lemon peel and juice, cannellini beans, carrots, tomatoes, olive oil, parsley, and pepper. Gently stir in tuna and serve.

Each serving: About 411 calories ▪ 36 g protein ▪ 49 g carbohydrate ▪ 11 g fiber ▪ 8 g total fat (1 g saturated) ▪ 25 mg cholesterol ▪ 306 mg sodium.

Waldorf Salad with turkey (6 g fiber)
Have 1 serving of salad with 3 ounces skinless turkey breast.

▶ Waldorf Salad
Prep: 20 minutes ■ Makes 6 servings

1 medium lemon
½ cup reduced-calorie mayonnaise
¼ teaspoon celery salt
¼ teaspoon ground white pepper
¼ teaspoon ground cardamom or cinnamon
2 large McIntosh apples
2 large pears
8 ounces seedless green or red grapes
2 cups sliced celery hearts, with leaves
1 bunch watercress
⅔ cup crumbled Stilton or Gorgonzola cheese
⅔ cup coarsely chopped black walnuts or filberts, toasted

1. Into large bowl, squeeze juice from lemon; stir in mayonnaise, celery salt, pepper, and cardamom.
2. Core and cut unpeeled apples and pears into 1-inch chunks; cut each grape in half.
3. Stir apples, pears, grapes, and celery into mixture. Cover bowl and refrigerate.
4. To serve, line platter with watercress. Stir cheese and walnuts into salad; spoon salad over watercress.
Each serving: About 307 calories ■ 7 g protein ■ 36 g carbohydrate ■ 6 g fiber ■ 18 g total fat (4 g saturated) 16 mg cholesterol ■ 402 mg sodium.

SANDWICHES/BURRITOS
Chicken Salad Sandwich with broccoli (5 g fiber)
Serve one fourth of the chicken salad between 2 slices of whole-wheat bread. Add 1 cup steamed or fresh broccoli tossed with a dash of balsamic vinegar.

▶ Chicken Salad

Prep: 20 minutes (plus cooling if you make chicken yourself) ▪ Cook: none if you use a rotisserie chicken (1 hour if you boil it yourself) ▪ Makes 4 servings

1 chicken (3 pounds) or 3 cups bite-size pieces cooked rotisserie
   chicken or turkey (without skin)
1½ teaspoons salt or ½ teaspoon if using rotisserie chicken
3 stalks celery, finely chopped
⅓ cup reduced-fat mayonnaise
2 teaspoons fresh lemon juice
¼ teaspoon black pepper

1. If you boil the chicken yourself: In a 4-quart saucepan, combine chicken, 1 teaspoon salt, and enough *water to cover;* heat to boiling over high heat. Reduce heat; cover and simmer gently until chicken loses its pink color throughout, about 45 minutes. Let stand another 30 minutes; drain (reserve broth for another use). When chicken is cool enough to handle, discard skin and bones; cut meat into bite-size pieces.

2. In medium bowl, combine celery, mayonnaise, lemon juice, remaining ½ teaspoon salt, and pepper; stir until blended. Add chicken and toss to coat.

Each serving (without bread): About 253 calories ▪ 31 g protein ▪ 5 g carbohydrate ▪ 1 g fiber ▪ 12 g total fat (3 g saturated) 98 mg cholesterol ▪ 800 mg sodium.

Classic Tuna Salad Sandwich with carrots and celery (7 g fiber)

Spread 1 serving Classic Tuna Salad (recipe, page 55) between 2 slices whole-wheat bread. Serve with 1 cup carrot and celery sticks and 2 tablespoons light ranch dressing on the side for dipping.

▶ Health Club Sandwiches (11 g fiber)

Have 1 sandwich.

Prep: 25 minutes ▪ Cook: 2 minutes ▪ Makes 4 sandwiches

2 tablespoons olive oil
2 teaspoons plus 1 tablespoon fresh lemon juice
1 teaspoon honey
⅛ teaspoon ground black pepper
3 carrots, peeled and shredded (1 cup)
2 cups alfalfa sprouts
1 garlic clove, finely chopped
½ teaspoon ground cumin
pinch ground red pepper (cayenne)
1 can (15 to 19 ounces) garbanzo beans, rinsed and drained
1 tablespoon water
8 slices whole-wheat bread, toasted
1 large ripe tomato (12 ounces), thinly sliced
1 bunch watercress, tough stems trimmed

1. In medium bowl, stir 1 tablespoon oil, 2 teaspoons lemon juice, honey, and black pepper until mixed. Add carrots and alfalfa sprouts; toss until evenly coated with dressing.

2. In a 2-quart saucepan, heat remaining 1 tablespoon oil over medium heat. Add garlic, cumin, and red pepper and cook until very fragrant. Stir in garbanzo beans and remove from heat. Add remaining 1 tablespoon lemon juice and water; mash to a coarse puree.

3. Spread 8 toast slices with garbanzo-bean mixture. Top 4 slices with tomato slices and watercress. Top remaining 4 slices with alfalfa sprout mixture and place on watercress-topped bread.

Each sandwich: About 380 calories ▪ 13 g protein ▪ 61 g carbohydrate ▪ 11 g fiber ▪ 11 g total fat (2 g saturated) ▪ 0 mg cholesterol ▪ 696 mg sodium.

▶ Hummus Sandwich (13 g fiber)

Spoon *⅓ cup store-bought hummus* into a *6-inch whole-wheat pita* with *1 slice reduced-fat Cheddar* and a *few tomato slices.* Serve with remaining tomato slices.

Or, make your own hummus (recipe, page 68).

▶ Peanut Butter and Jelly Sandwich (7 g fiber)

Spread *4 teaspoons peanut butter* and *2 teaspoons jam or jelly* on *2 slices of whole-wheat bread.*

Serve with 1 cup fat-free milk and ½ cup carrots.

Smoked Salmon Sandwich with salad (6 g fiber)

Serve the sandwich with a green salad: 1½ cups *each* watercress and romaine tossed with 1 tablespoon vinaigrette and topped with 6 almonds.

▶ Smoked Salmon Sandwich

Prep: 15 minutes ▪ Makes 1 serving

2 tablespoons reduced-fat cream cheese, softened
1 scant teaspoon minced shallot
1 scant teaspoon capers, drained and chopped
1 scant teaspoon chopped fresh dill plus additional sprig
1 spritz fresh lemon juice
2 slices pumpernickel bread
2 ounces thinly sliced smoked salmon
ground black pepper to taste
1 teaspoon salmon caviar (optional)
dill sprigs

In small bowl, stir cream cheese, shallot, capers, chopped dill, and lemon juice until well blended. Spread mixture evenly on 1 slice bread. Top with smoked salmon slices. Sprinkle lightly with pepper. Sprinkle on caviar, if you like, and top with dill sprigs and the remaining slice of bread.

Each sandwich: About 282 calories ▪ 20 g protein ▪ 28 g carbohydrate ▪ 3 g fiber ▪ 10 g total fat (4 g saturated) ▪ 61 mg cholesterol ▪ 1728 mg sodium.

Turkey and Swiss Sandwich with salad (8 g fiber)

Serve the sandwich with a salad: 2 cups mixed greens and the remaining tomato tossed with 1 teaspoon olive oil, vinegar or lemon juice, and salt and pepper to taste.

At Subway: Have a turkey sandwich and 2 servings of Swiss cheese on an "Atkins-Friendly Wrap." Also have a garden salad with ⅓ packet of Fat-Free Wine Vinaigrette dressing (14 g fiber).

▶ Turkey and Swiss Sandwich

Layer *2 ounces (about 2 thick slices) turkey breast* and *1 ounce (about 1 sandwich-size slice) Swiss cheese* between *2 slices whole-wheat bread.*

Vegetarian Black Bean Burrito with crudités (15 g fiber)

Serve 1 homemade burrito or a Taco Bell Bean Burrito (11 g fiber with crudités) with 1 cup of crudités (e.g., cauliflower, celery, cherry tomatoes) dipped in 1½ tablespoons light ranch dressing.

▶ Vegetarian Black Bean Burrito

Prep: 10 minutes ▪ Cook: 15 minutes ▪ Makes 4 servings

> 4 (8-inch) low-fat tortillas, preferably whole-wheat, no more than 130 calories each
> 1¼ cups corn kernels cut from cobs (about 2 large ears) or use frozen, thawed, or no-sodium added canned
> 1 can (15 ounces) spicy fat-free black bean chili
> 1 can (8 ounces) tomato sauce, preferably reduced-sodium
> ½ cup shredded Monterey Jack cheese with jalapeño chiles
> ⅓ cup packed fresh cilantro leaves, chopped

1. Preheat the oven to 300°F. Wrap tortillas in foil; heat in oven until warm, about 15 minutes.

2. In medium saucepan, stir corn, chili, and tomato sauce. Heat to boiling over medium-high heat; boil 1 minute.

3. Spoon about 1 cup chili mixture down center of each tortilla; sprinkle with cheese and cilantro. Fold opposite sides of tortilla over filling. Place burritos seam side down on platter and serve.

Each burrito: About 347 calories ▪ 15 g protein ▪ 54 g carbohydrate ▪ 14 g fiber ▪ 9 g total fat (3 g saturated) ▪ 13 mg cholesterol ▪ 843 mg sodium.

Vegetarian Burger with salad (13 g fiber)
Serve 1 burger and salsa with a chopped salad: ½ cup *each* diced tomatoes and green pepper tossed with ½ teaspoon olive oil, 1 spritz lemon juice, and salt and pepper to taste.

▶ Vegetarian Burger with Avocado Salsa
Prep: 10 minutes ▪ Cook: As label directs ▪ Makes 4 servings

   1 medium-size avocado
   1 green onion, chopped
   2 tablespoons bottled mild salsa
   1 tablespoon lemon juice
   1 tablespoon chopped fresh cilantro
   ¼ teaspoon salt
   2 packages (6.35 ounces each) refrigerated vegetarian soy
      burgers (4 burgers)
   4 sandwich rolls, split
   1 large tomato
   4 large lettuce leaves
   1 cup alfalfa sprouts

1. Preheat broiler if manufacturer directs. Cut avocado lengthwise in half; remove seed and peel. In bowl, mash avocado; stir in green onion, salsa, lemon juice, cilantro, and salt.
2. Cook vegetarian soy burgers as label directs. Meanwhile, toast sandwich rolls and slice tomato.
3. On 4 dinner plates, arrange lettuce leaves on bottom halves of toasted rolls; top with tomato slices, burgers, and avocado mixture. Replace tops. Serve with alfalfa sprouts.
Each sandwich: About 328 calories ▪ 20 g protein ▪ 36 g carbohydrate ▪ 10 g fiber ▪ 14 g total fat (2 g saturated) ▪ 0 mg cholesterol ▪ 707 mg sodium.

SOUPS
▶ Entire-Meal Tomato Soup (12 g fiber)
Prep: 5 minutes ▪ Cook: 5 minutes ▪ Makes 1 serving

1½ cups tomato soup, preferably reduced-sodium
2 tablespoons dry couscous, preferably whole-wheat
½ cup canned white beans or garbanzo beans, rinsed and drained
3 cups fresh spinach
1 tablespoon fresh lemon juice
2 tablespoons feta cheese or goat cheese

In medium saucepan, heat tomato soup to boiling. Add couscous and beans. Reduce heat and simmer 3 minutes. Add spinach; simmer another 2 minutes. Remove from heat and stir in lemon juice. Serve with cheese crumbled on top.

Each serving (using reduced-sodium tomato soup): About 402 calories ■ 18 g protein ■ 68 g carbohydrate ■ 12 g fiber ■ 9 g total fat (3 g saturated) ■ 17 mg cholesterol ■ 394 mg sodium.

Italian White Bean and Spinach Soup with crackers (16 g fiber)
Serve 1 serving of the soup with about ½ ounce crackers, preferably whole-wheat (check label for 70 calories' worth).

▶ Italian White Bean and Spinach Soup (16 g fiber)
Prep: 20 minutes ■ Cook: 30 minutes ■ Makes about 4 servings (7½ cups).

1 tablespoon canola oil
1 medium onion, chopped
1 stalk celery, chopped
1 garlic clove, finely chopped
2 cans (15 to 19 ounces each) white kidney beans (cannellini),
    rinsed and drained
2 cups water
1 can (14½ ounces) reduced-sodium chicken broth or 1¾ cups
    homemade or from a carton
¼ teaspoon ground black pepper
⅛ teaspoon dried thyme
1 bunch (10 to 12 ounces) spinach, tough stems trimmed
1 tablespoon lemon juice
Freshly grated Parmesan cheese (optional)

1. In 3-quart saucepan, heat oil over medium heat. Add onion and celery; cook, stirring, until celery is tender, 5 to 8 minutes. Stir in garlic and cook 30 seconds. Add beans, water, broth, pepper, and thyme; heat to boiling over high heat. Reduce heat and simmer 15 minutes.

2. Roll up several spinach leaves together, cigar fashion, and cut crosswise into thin slices. Repeat with remaining spinach.

3. With slotted spoon, remove 2 cups beans from soup mixture and reserve. Spoon one-fourth of mixture into blender; cover, with center part of cover removed to let steam escape, and puree until smooth. Pour puree into bowl. Repeat with remaining mixture.

4. Return puree and reserved beans to saucepan; heat to boiling over medium-high heat. Stir in spinach and cook just until wilted, about 1 minute. Remove from heat and stir in lemon juice. Top each serving with 1 tablespoon grated Parmesan, if you like.

Each serving (scant 2 cups): About 334 calories ▪ 20 g protein ▪ 57 g carbohydrate ▪ 14 g fiber ▪ 5 g total fat (0 g saturated) ▪ 0 mg cholesterol ▪ 132 mg sodium.

Black bean soup with cheese and crackers (17 g fiber)

Heat 1½ cups canned black bean soup (about 250 calories). Add 3 cups fresh spinach or arugula or other leafy green of your choice and simmer a few minutes. Serve with a few whole-grain crackers (about 25 calories) and 1 slice (1 ounce) reduced-fat Cheddar or Swiss.

500-Calorie Dinners

BEEF AND PORK

Burger and "fries" (5 g fiber)

Prepare burger and fries (below). Place the burger on half a whole-grain hamburger roll, spread with mustard, if desired, and top with slices of lettuce and tomato. (Discard the other half bun, or use it in another meal.) Using sweet potatoes instead of white potatoes for the fries gives you a big nutrition advantage: five times the vitamin A requirement versus no vitamin A in the white potato.

Have the remainder of the tomato, sliced, on the side. (If you make the recipe for four servings, use 3 medium tomatoes. If making one serving just for yourself, use a smallish tomato.)

▶ Classic Hamburgers
Prep: 5 minutes ▪ Cook: 8 minutes ▪ Makes 4 burgers

    1¼ pounds ground round (85% lean)
    ½ teaspoon salt
    ¼ teaspoon ground black pepper

1. Shape ground beef into 4 patties, each ¾ inch thick, handling meat as little as possible. Sprinkle patties with salt and pepper.

2. Heat 12-inch skillet over high heat until hot but not smoking. Add patties and cook about 4 minutes per side for medium or until desired doneness.

Each burger: About 284 calories ▪ 29 g protein ▪ 0 g carbohydrate ▪ 0 g fiber ▪ 18 g total fat (7 g saturated) ▪ 102 mg cholesterol ▪ 372 mg sodium.

▶ Oven Fries
Prep: 10 minutes ▪ Bake: 45 minutes ▪ Makes 4 servings

    3 medium sweet potatoes or baking potatoes (about 6 ounces
        each), not peeled
    1 tablespoon canola or olive oil
    ½ teaspoon salt
    ⅛ teaspoon pepper

1. Preheat oven to 425°F. Cut each potato lengthwise into quarters, then cut each quarter lengthwise into 3 wedges.

2. Place potatoes in 15½ by 10½-inch jelly-roll pan. Add oil, salt, and pepper; toss until potatoes are evenly coated. Bake, turning occasionally, until tender, about 45 minutes.

Each serving (using sweet potatoes): About 170 calories ▪ 2 g protein ▪ 33 g carbohydrate ▪ 4 g fiber ▪ 4 g total fat (0 g saturated) ▪ 0 mg cholesterol ▪ 304 mg sodium.

Filet Mignon with Tomatoes and Roquefort (6 g fiber)

Have 1 serving with a 3-ounce glass of wine (or have an extra slice of French bread).

Prep: 15 minutes ■ Cook: 20 minutes ■ Makes 4 servings

2 large tomatoes (about 1 pound)

12 ounces French green beans (haricots verts) or green beans, trimmed

2 tablespoons light, trans fat–free corn-oil spread

8 ounces oyster or regular mushrooms, sliced

2 teaspoons reduced-sodium soy sauce

½ cup water

¾ teaspoon cornstarch

½ teaspoon reduced-sodium beef-flavor instant bouillon

4 beef tenderloin steaks (filet mignon), each 1 inch thick (4 ounces each)

½ teaspoon salt

2 tablespoons white wine (optional)

1 ounce Roquefort or blue cheese, crumbled (about ¼ cup)

1 loaf (8 ounces) French or Italian bread

1. Cut center part of each tomato into two ¾-inch-thick slices; reserve ends for another use.

2. In 4-quart saucepan, heat *1 inch water* to boiling over high heat. Add green beans; heat to boiling. Reduce heat to low; cover and simmer until beans are tender-crisp, 5 to 8 minutes. Drain beans and place in bowl.

3. In same saucepan, heat 2 teaspoons light corn-oil spread over medium-high heat until hot. Add mushrooms and cook, stirring frequently, until golden. Add green beans and soy sauce; keep warm.

4. In cup, mix water, cornstarch, and beef bouillon until blended; set aside.

5. In nonstick 12-inch skillet, heat remaining 1 teaspoon light corn-oil spread over medium-high heat until hot. Add steaks, season with salt, and cook, turning steaks once, about 10 minutes for medium-rare or until desired doneness. Transfer steaks to plates; keep warm.

6. In same skillet, cook tomatoes, turning once, just until hot. Transfer to 4 warm dinner plates.

7. Add wine to skillet, if using; cook, stirring, 30 seconds. Stir in cornstarch mixture; cook until sauce thickens slightly, about 1 minute. Top each tomato slice with a steak. Spoon sauce over steaks; sprinkle steaks with crumbled Roquefort cheese. Serve steaks with green-bean mixture and bread.

Each serving: About 435 calories ■ 35 g protein ■ 44 g carbohydrate ■ 7 g fiber ■ 15 g total fat (5 g saturated) ■ 78 mg cholesterol ■ 997 mg sodium.

Orange-Glazed Steak with Pear and Blue Cheese Salad and Sweet Potato (6 g fiber)

Have 1 serving of steak with the salad and half a baked sweet potato. To bake a sweet potato: Puncture with a fork in two places and bake at 400°F for 40 minutes. Or boil until soft, or microwave on high for 5 to 6 minutes and let rest for 1 minute.

❯ Pear and Blue Cheese Salad

Toss *2 cups mixed greens, ½ diced pear,* and *2 tablespoons crumbled blue cheese,* with *1 teaspoon olive oil* and *½ teaspoon vinegar.*

❯ Orange-Glazed Steak

Prep: 5 minutes plus marinating ■ Cook: 5 minutes ■ Makes 6 servings

¼ cup soy sauce
2 garlic cloves, crushed with garlic press
1 teaspoon coarsely ground black pepper
1 top round steak, 1¼ inches thick (about 2 pounds)
⅓ cup orange marmalade

1. In 13″ by 9″ glass baking dish, mix soy sauce, garlic, and pepper. Trim fat from round steak; add steak to soy sauce mixture, turning to coat. Cover and refrigerate 30 minutes, turning once.

2. Meanwhile, prepare grill.

3. Place steak on grill rack over medium heat; spoon remaining marinade over steak. Grill, turning steak occasionally, 25 minutes for medium-rare or until desired doneness, brushing with orange marmalade during last 10 minutes of grilling.

4. Transfer steak to cutting board and let stand 10 minutes to set juices for easier slicing. Cut into thin slices across the grain.

Each serving: About 271 calories ▪ 41 g protein ▪ 12 g carbohydrate ▪ 0 g fiber ▪ 6 g total fat (2 g saturated) ▪ 102 mg cholesterol ▪ 161 mg sodium.

Pork Steak with Plum Glaze and Lemon-Parsley Rice with zucchini (5 g fiber)

Serve the steak and rice with ½ cup grilled zucchini. To grill zucchini: Brush 1 cup zucchini slices with ½ teaspoon olive oil. Grill zucchini along with the pork; it will shrink to about ½ cup cooked.

▌ Pork Steak with Plum Glaze

Prep: 10 minutes ▪ Grill: 6 minutes ▪ Makes 4 servings

1 pork tenderloin (about 1 pound)
1 teaspoon salt
¼ teaspoon coarsely ground black pepper
½ cup plum jam or preserves
1 tablespoon brown sugar
1 tablespoon grated peeled fresh ginger
1 tablespoon fresh lemon juice
½ teaspoon ground cinnamon
2 garlic cloves, crushed with garlic press
4 large plums (about 1 pound), each cut in half and pitted

1. Prepare grill. Cut pork tenderloin lengthwise, almost in half, being careful not to cut all the way through. Open up like a book and spread flat. With meat mallet or rolling pin, between two sheets plastic wrap or waxed paper, pound tenderloin to about ¼-inch thickness. Cut the tenderloin into 4 pieces; season with salt and pepper.

2. In small bowl, mix plum jam, brown sugar, ginger, lemon juice, cinnamon, and garlic. Brush one side of each pork steak and cut side of each plum half with plum-jam glaze. Place pork and plums, glaze side down, on hot grill rack over medium heat and grill 3 minutes. Brush steaks and plums with remaining glaze; turn and grill until steaks are lightly browned on both sides and just lose their pink color throughout and plums are hot, about 3 minutes longer.

Each serving: About 309 calories ■ 25 g protein ■ 42 g carbohydrate ■ 2 g fiber ■ 5 g total fat (1 g saturated) ■ 66 mg cholesterol ■ 524 mg sodium.

▶ Lemon-Parsley Rice
Prep: 5 minutes ■ Cook: 40 minutes (5 minutes if using instant brown rice) ■ Makes 4 servings

    1 cup low-sodium chicken broth
    1 cup water
    1 cup brown rice
    ¼ teaspoon salt
    2 tablespoons chopped parsley
    1 teaspoon grated lemon peel

1. In a 3-quart saucepan, heat broth and water to boiling over high heat. Stir in rice and salt; heat to boiling. Reduce heat to low; cover and simmer, without stirring or lifting lid, until rice is tender and all liquid has been absorbed, 40 to 45 minutes.

2. Remove pan from heat and let stand 5 minutes.

3. To serve, fluff rice with fork. Stir in parsley and lemon peel.

Each serving: About 175 calories ■ 4 g protein ■ 36 g carbohydrate ■ 2 g fiber ■ 1 g total fat (0 g saturated) ■ 0 mg cholesterol ■ 175 mg sodium.

CHICKEN
Chicken Caesar Salad with sweet potato (9 g fiber)
Serve the salad with a large sweet potato dressed with 2 tablespoons reduced-fat sour cream. To bake a sweet potato: Puncture with a fork in two places and bake at 400°F for 40 minutes. Or boil until soft, or microwave on high for 5 to 6 minutes and let rest for 1 minute.

▶ Chicken Caesar Salad

Prep: 10 minutes ▪ Cook: 5 minutes ▪ Makes 4 servings

12 ounces chicken-breast tenders
1 tablespoon canola oil
1 bag (7½ to 10 ounces) regular or reduced-fat Caesar salad kit
    (e.g., Earthbound Farms)
1 bag (5 ounces) baby romaine or baby spinach leaves
¾ cup matchstick-thin carrots
⅛ teaspoon coarsely ground black pepper

1. Heat ridged grill pan or heavy 10-inch skillet over medium-high heat until hot but not smoking.

2. Meanwhile, in medium bowl, toss chicken with oil.

3. Add chicken to grill pan or skillet and cook, turning once, just until chicken loses its pink color throughout, 4 to 5 minutes.

4. While chicken is cooking, in large bowl, toss lettuce, dressing, croutons, and Parmesan from Caesar salad kit with romaine and carrots.

5. Add chicken to salad, sprinkle with pepper, and toss again.

Each serving: About 259 calories ▪ 16 g protein ▪ 21 g carbohydrate ▪ 3 g fiber ▪ 13 g total fat (2 g saturated) ▪ 35 mg cholesterol ▪ 559 mg sodium.

Chicken with couscous and spinach (11 g fiber)

Toss one sixth of the couscous recipe with ⅓ cup cooked skinless chicken breast strips (pull them off a rotisserie chicken breast or use the precooked Tyson Chicken Breast Strips or Perdue Short Cuts, or make your own). Serve with 1 serving Garlicky Spinach.

▶ Jeweled Cinnamon Couscous

Prep: 5 minutes ▪ Cook: 10 minutes ▪ Makes 6 servings (8 cups)

1 tablespoon trans fat–free margarine or butter
½ medium red onion, chopped
1 package (8 ounces) sliced mushrooms
1 can (14 to 14½ ounces) low-sodium vegetable broth
¼ cup water

1 can (15 to 19 ounces) low-sodium garbanzo beans
½ cup dried cranberries
½ cup golden raisins
¼ cup dry sherry
1 teaspoon salt
½ teaspoon ground cinnamon
¼ teaspoon ground black pepper
1 package (10 ounces) plain couscous

1. In deep 12-inch skillet, melt margarine over medium-high heat. Add onion and mushrooms; cook, stirring occasionally, 3 minutes.

2. Meanwhile, in 1-quart saucepan, heat broth and water to boiling over high heat.

3. Stir beans, cranberries, raisins, sherry, salt, cinnamon, and pepper into mushroom mixture. Remove skillet from heat.

4. Add couscous to skillet; stir in hot broth. Cover and let mixture stand 5 minutes or until liquid is absorbed. Fluff with fork before serving.

Each serving (about 1⅓ cups): About 367 calories ■ 12 g protein ■ 71 g carbohydrate ■ 7 g fiber ■ 3 g total fat (0 g saturated) ■ 0 mg cholesterol ■ 512 mg sodium.

▌ Garlicky Spinach
Prep: 5 minutes ■ Cook: 5 minutes ■ Makes 4 servings

1 tablespoon olive oil
1 large garlic clove, minced
2 bags (10 ounces each) fresh spinach, rinsed and drained but
   not spun dry, tough stems trimmed
¼ teaspoon salt

In 12-inch skillet, heat oil over medium-high heat until hot. Add garlic and cook, stirring, until fragrant, about 30 seconds. Stir in half the spinach with water clinging to leaves; cover and cook just until wilted, about 2 minutes. Add remaining spinach and cook, uncovered, until tender, about 2 minutes longer. Stir in salt.

Each serving: About 60 calories ▪ 4 g protein ▪ 5 g carbohydrate ▪ 4 g fiber ▪ 4 g total fat (1 g saturated) ▪ 0 mg cholesterol ▪ 249 mg sodium.

Rotisserie chicken with sweet potato and Roasted Cauliflower (7 g fiber)

Have either a chicken leg (no skin) or half a breast (no skin) and a medium sweet potato. To bake a sweet potato: Puncture with a fork in two places and bake at 400°F for 40 minutes. Or boil until soft, or microwave on high for 5 to 6 minutes and let rest for 1 minute.

▶ Roasted Cauliflower

Prep: 10 minutes ▪ Roast: 23 minutes ▪ Makes 4 servings

> 1 medium head cauliflower (about 2 pounds), cut into ¾-inch
>   pieces
> 1 tablespoon olive oil
> ½ teaspoon salt
> ¼ teaspoon coarsely ground black pepper
> 2 tablespoons chopped fresh parsley
> 1 garlic clove, finely chopped

1. Preheat oven to 450°F. In jelly-roll pan, toss cauliflower with oil, salt, and pepper until cauliflower is evenly coated. Roast until cauliflower is tender, stirring halfway through roasting, about 20 minutes.

2. In small cup, combine parsley and garlic. Sprinkle over cauliflower and stir until evenly mixed. Roast 3 minutes longer.

Each serving: About 68 calories ▪ 3 g protein ▪ 8 g carbohydrate ▪ 4 g fiber ▪ 4 g total fat (1 g saturated) ▪ 0 mg cholesterol ▪ 335 mg sodium.

Texas Chicken Burger with broccoli (13 g fiber)

Serve 1 burger with 1 cup steamed broccoli drizzled with 1 teaspoon olive oil, a spritz of lemon juice, and salt and pepper to taste.

▶ Texas Chicken Burgers

Prep: 20 minutes plus standing ▪ Cook: 10 minutes ▪ Makes 4 burgers

1 pound ground chicken meat
2 green onions, chopped
1 small zucchini (about 5 ounces), grated
1 medium-size carrot, grated
1 tablespoon chili powder
¾ teaspoon salt
¼ teaspoon ground cumin
⅛ teaspoon ground red pepper (cayenne)
1 can (16 ounces) vegetarian baked beans
1 tablespoon prepared mustard
1 tablespoon light molasses
4 whole-grain sandwich rolls, each cut horizontally in half
lettuce leaves

1. In medium bowl, combine ground chicken, green onions, zucchini, carrot, chili powder, salt, cumin, and ground red pepper just until well blended but not overmixed.

2. On waxed paper, shape mixture into four 3½-inch round patties, pressing firmly; set aside.

3. In 1-quart saucepan over medium heat, heat beans, mustard, and molasses to boiling.

4. Meanwhile, spray heavy 12-inch skillet with nonstick cooking spray. Heat skillet over medium-high heat until very hot but not smoking. Add patties to hot skillet and cook 5 minutes. Turn patties and cook until no longer pink inside (internal temperature should reach 165°F), about 5 minutes longer.

5. Top bottom half of each roll with lettuce, then with a patty. Replace tops of rolls. Serve with baked beans.

Each burger (with 4 ounces beans): About 429 calories ▪ 34 g protein ▪ 51 g carbohydrate ▪ 10 g fiber ▪ 10 g total fat (3 g saturated) ▪ 92 mg cholesterol ▪ 1,037 mg sodium.

FISH AND SHELLFISH
Grilled Halibut with grilled vegetables and beer (8 g fiber)
Along with the fish, grill 1 ear of corn (about 8 inches), husk and silk removed (about ¾ cup cooked corn kernels) seasoned with 2 teaspoons

of trans fat–free margarine and salt and pepper to taste. Add a portobello mushroom cap and half a red pepper drizzled with 1 teaspoon olive oil.

Have 1 serving of the fish and the grilled vegetables; enjoy with 8 ounces of light beer or 4 ounces of juice mixed with seltzer or something else for 65 calories.

▶ Grilled Halibut with Fresh Dill
Prep: 5 minutes plus marinating ▪ Grill: 10 minutes ▪ Makes 4 servings

¼ cup Worcestershire sauce for chicken
2 tablespoons fresh lemon juice
1 tablespoon olive oil
1 tablespoon minced fresh dill
¼ teaspoon coarsely ground black pepper
2 halibut steaks, 1 inch thick (about 12 ounces each)

1. In medium bowl, stir Worcestershire, lemon juice, oil, dill, and pepper. Place halibut in large ziptight plastic bag; add Worcestershire mixture. Seal bag, pressing out excess air, and place on plate. Refrigerate at least 2 hours, turning bag once.
2. Prepare grill. Place halibut on hot grill rack over low heat, reserving marinade. Cook, turning occasionally and basting frequently with reserved marinade, until opaque throughout, about 10 minutes. Cut steaks in half and serve.

Safety tip: Make sure that fish cooks after final addition of marinade. In other words, don't add marinade once fish is removed from grill, since it was basting the raw fish.
Each serving: About 197 calories ▪ 33 g protein ▪ 2 g carbohydrate ▪ 0 g fiber ▪ 5 g total fat (1 g saturated) ▪ 51 mg cholesterol ▪ 188 mg sodium.

Honey-Lime Salmon with salad and garlic bread (4 g fiber)
Have 1 salmon fillet with a chopped salad (¾ cup *each* chopped tomato and cucumber mixed with 1 teaspoon olive oil, and vinegar, salt, and pepper to taste) and garlic bread (medium slice whole-grain, crusty

bread spread with a mix of half teaspoon olive oil, ½ clove crushed garlic, and pepper/red pepper flakes to taste). Grill the garlic bread alongside the salmon.

▶ Honey-Lime Salmon

Prep: 10 minutes ▪ Grill: 10 minutes ▪ Makes 4 servings

3 tablespoons honey
1 teaspoon very hot water
1 teaspoon ground cumin
1 teaspoon ground coriander
¾ teaspoon grated fresh lime peel
¾ teaspoon salt
¼ teaspoon coarsely ground black pepper
4 pieces salmon fillet, ¾-inch thick (about 6 ounces each), skin
    removed
3 tablespoons chopped fresh cilantro leaves
lime wedges

1. In cup, mix honey, hot water, cumin, coriander, lime peel, salt, and pepper until blended.

2. With tweezers, remove any bones from salmon. Rub honey-spice mixture over fillets.

3. Prepare grill. Place salmon on lightly oiled grill rack and cook over medium heat 4 minutes. With wide metal spatula, carefully turn salmon over; cook until just opaque throughout, 4 to 5 minutes longer.

4. Sprinkle salmon with cilantro and serve with lime wedges.

Tip: You can substitute red snapper or bluefish fillets for the salmon.

Each serving: About 342 calories ▪ 32 g protein ▪ 11 g carbohydrate ▪ 0 g fiber ▪ 18 g total fat (4 g saturated) ▪ 91 mg cholesterol ▪ 487 mg sodium.

Scallops with Watercress, with Bulgur Wheat (5 g fiber)

Have one serving scallops with ¾ cup cooked Bulgur Wheat or cooked brown rice.

▶ Scallops with Watercress

Prep: 10 minutes ▪ Cook: 10 minutes ▪ Makes 4 servings

1½ pounds sea scallops
3 tablespoons olive oil
⅛ teaspoon ground black pepper
¾ teaspoon salt
2 bunches watercress, tough stems trimmed
2 tablespoons water
1 tablespoon fresh lemon juice
1 tablespoon capers, drained and chopped
2 tablespoons butter (do not use margarine)

1. Rinse scallops with cold running water. Pull off and discard tough crescent-shaped muscle from each scallop. Pat scallops dry with paper towels. Cut each scallop horizontally in half if large.

2. In 10-inch skillet, heat 1 tablespoon oil over medium-high heat. Add scallops, pepper, and ½ teaspoon salt and cook, stirring, until just opaque throughout and lightly golden, about 5 minutes.

3. Meanwhile, in 5-quart Dutch oven or saucepot, heat remaining 2 tablespoons oil over high heat. Add watercress and remaining ¼ teaspoon salt and cook, stirring, just until watercress wilts, about 2 minutes. Divide watercress among 4 warm plates; top with scallops.

4. In same skillet, heat water, lemon juice, and capers to boiling over medium-high heat. Reduce heat to medium; add butter, 1 tablespoon at a time, beating with a wire whisk just until butter has melted and mixture thickens. Pour sauce over scallops.

Each serving: About 304 calories ▪ 25 g protein ▪ 5 g carbohydrate ▪ 0 g fiber ▪ 21 g total fat (5 g saturated) ▪ 62 mg cholesterol ▪ 375 mg sodium.

▶ Bulgur Wheat
Prep: 1 minute ▪ Cook: 15 minutes ▪ Makes 2½ servings (about 2 cups)

1 cup cracked wheat or coarse bulgur wheat
1⅔ cup reduced-sodium chicken or vegetable broth

In medium saucepan, combine bulgur wheat and broth and heat to boiling over medium-high heat, stirring occasionally. Reduce heat; cover and simmer until liquid has been absorbed, 15 to 20 minutes.

Each serving (¾ cup): About 186 calories ▪ 7 g protein ▪ 41 g carbohydrate ▪ 10 g fiber ▪ 1 g total fat (0 g saturated) ▪ 0 mg cholesterol ▪ 71 mg sodium.

Snapper Livornese with Lemon-Parsley Rice and broccoli (7 g fiber)

Have 1 serving of the snapper with 1 serving of Lemon-Parsley Rice (page 106) and 1 cup steamed broccoli seasoned with a spritz of lemon juice.

▶ Snapper Livornese

Vibrant with olives, capers, and basil, this preparation works beautifully with any lean white fish.

Prep: 10 minutes ▪ Cook: 25 minutes ▪ Makes 4 servings

> 1 tablespoon olive oil
> 1 garlic clove, finely chopped
> 1 can (14 to 16 ounces) tomatoes
> 1/8 teaspoon salt
> 1/8 teaspoon ground black pepper
> 4 red snapper fillets (6 ounces each)
> 1/4 cup chopped fresh basil
> 1/4 cup Kalamata or Gaeta olives, pitted and chopped
> 2 teaspoons capers, drained

1. In nonstick 10-inch skillet, heat oil over medium heat. Add garlic and cook just until very fragrant, about 30 seconds. Stir in tomatoes with their juice, salt, and pepper, breaking up tomatoes with side of spoon. Heat to boiling; reduce heat and simmer 10 minutes.

2. With tweezers, remove any bones from snapper fillets. Place fillets, skin side down, in skillet. Cover and simmer until fish is just opaque throughout, about 10 minutes. With wide slotted spatula, transfer fish to warm platter. Stir basil, olives, and capers into tomato sauce and spoon over snapper.

Each serving: About 255 calories ▪ 38 g protein ▪ 6 g carbohydrate ▪ 1 g fiber ▪ 8 g total fat (1 g saturated) ▪ 67 mg cholesterol ▪ 797 mg sodium.

Tuscan Tuna Salad Pita with salad (8 g fiber)
Serve 1 pita with a feta-topped salad: 2 cups mixed greens; 1 cup chopped vegetables, such as tomatoes and mushrooms; 1 tablespoon oil/vinegar dressing; 2 tablespoons feta.

▶ **Tuscan Tuna Salad Pita Sandwiches** (8 g fiber)
Prep: 15 minutes ▪ Makes 4 servings

   1 can (15 to 19 ounces) white kidney beans (cannellini), rinsed
      and drained
   ½ cup chopped fresh basil
   3 tablespoons capers, drained and chopped
   2 tablespoons fresh lemon juice
   2 tablespoons olive oil
   ¼ teaspoon coarsely ground black pepper
   1 can (6 ounces) light tuna packed in water, drained and flaked
   1 bunch watercress (4 ounces), tough stems trimmed and sprigs
      cut in half
   4 (6½-inch) whole-wheat pita breads (170 calories each), each
      cut horizontally in half
   2 medium ripe tomatoes (12 ounces), thinly sliced

   1. In a large bowl, mash 1 cup beans. Stir in basil, capers, lemon juice, oil, and pepper until well blended. Add tuna, watercress, and remaining beans; toss to mix.
   2. Spoon one fourth of tuna mixture into each pita and stuff with tomato slices.
Each pita: About 391 calories ▪ 24 g protein ▪ 55 g carbohydrate ▪ 11 g fiber ▪ 10 g total fat (1.3 g saturated) ▪ 12 mg cholesterol ▪ 725 mg sodium.

PASTA AND RICE

Pad Thai with spinach (4 g fiber)
Have 1 serving of Pad Thai with ½ cup cooked spinach (3 cups raw, steamed or microwaved until wilted) tossed with a few drops of soy sauce and ½ teaspoon grated ginger, if desired.

▶ Pad Thai

Prep: 25 minutes plus soaking ▪ Cook: 5 minutes ▪ Makes 4 servings

> 1 package (7 to 8 ounces) rice stick noodles (rice vermicelli) or
>   8 ounces angel hair pasta
> ¼ cup fresh lime juice
> ¼ cup Asian fish sauce (nam pla)
> 2 tablespoons sugar
> 1 tablespoon peanut or canola oil
> 8 ounces medium shrimp, shelled, deveined, and cut lengthwise
>   in half
> 2 garlic cloves, finely chopped
> ¼ teaspoon crushed red pepper
> 3 large eggs, lightly beaten
> 6 ounces fresh bean sprouts (about 2 cups), rinsed and drained
> ¼ cup unsalted roasted peanuts, coarsely chopped
> 3 green onions, thinly sliced
> ½ cup loosely packed fresh cilantro leaves
> lime wedges

1. In large bowl, soak rice stick noodles, if using, in enough *hot water* to cover for 20 minutes; drain. With kitchen shears, cut noodles into 4-inch lengths. If using angel hair pasta, break in half, cook in large saucepot as label directs, then drain and rinse with cold running water.

2. Meanwhile, in small bowl, combine lime juice, fish sauce, and sugar. Assemble all remaining ingredients and place next to stove.

3. In 12-inch skillet, heat oil over high heat until hot. Add shrimp, garlic, and crushed red pepper; cook, stirring, 1 minute. Add eggs and cook, stirring, until just set, about 20 seconds. Add drained noodles and cook, stirring, 2 minutes. Add fish-sauce mixture, half of bean sprouts, half of peanuts, and half of green onions; cook, stirring, 1 minute.

4. Transfer Pad Thai to warm platter or serving bowl. Top with remaining bean sprouts, remaining peanuts, remaining green onions, and the cilantro. Serve with lime wedges.

Each serving: About 495 calories ▪ 25 g protein ▪ 65 g carbohydrate ▪ 2 g fiber ▪ 17 g total fat (3 g saturated) ▪ 235 mg cholesterol ▪ 827 mg sodium.

▶ **Penne with Salmon and Asparagus** (9 g fiber)
Have 1 serving.
Prep: 15 minutes ▪ Cook: 30 minutes ▪ Makes 6 servings

   1 package (16 ounces) penne rigate or bow ties, preferably
      whole-wheat
   3 teaspoons olive oil
   1½ pounds asparagus, trimmed and cut into 2-inch pieces
   ½ teaspoon salt
   ¼ teaspoon coarsely ground black pepper
   1 large shallot, finely chopped (¼ cup)
   ⅓ cup dry white wine
   1 cup low-sodium chicken broth
   1 or 2 skinless salmon fillets (1⅓ pounds), cut crosswise into
      thirds, then lengthwise into ¼-inch-thick slices
   1 tablespoon chopped fresh tarragon

   1. In large saucepot, cook pasta as label directs; drain.
   2. Meanwhile, in nonstick 12-inch skillet, heat 2 teaspoons oil over
medium-high heat. Add asparagus, salt, and pepper and cook until
asparagus is almost tender-crisp, about 5 minutes. Add shallot and
remaining 1 teaspoon oil; cook, stirring constantly, 2 minutes longer.
Add wine; heat to boiling over high heat. Stir in broth and heat to boiling. In single layer, arrange salmon slices in skillet; cover and cook until
just opaque throughout, 2 to 3 minutes. Remove skillet from heat; stir
in tarragon.
   3. In warm serving bowl, toss pasta with asparagus mixture.
Each serving: About 509 calories ▪ 32 g protein ▪ 59 g carbohydrate ▪ 9 g
fiber ▪ 16 g total fat (3 g saturated) ▪ 60 mg cholesterol ▪ 273 mg sodium.

Whole-wheat pasta with Marinara Sauce, with salad (13 g fiber)
Cook 1 heaping cup penne, rigatoni, or other short, tubular whole-
wheat pasta according to package directions. Drain and top with ½ cup
Marinara Sauce (bottled, or use recipe below) and 1 tablespoon freshly
grated Parmesan. Serve with arugula salad: 2 cups arugula or watercress
tossed with 1 teaspoon olive oil and lemon juice, salt and pepper to

taste. Add 2 ounces cooked chicken or shrimp to either the pasta or the salad. (You can cook raw shrimp in the simmering sauce for 3 to 5 minutes or until opaque throughout, but chicken must be precooked.)

▶ Marinara Sauce
Prep: 5 minutes ■ Cook: 30 minutes ■ Makes 6 servings (3½ cups)

> 2 tablespoon olive oil
> 1 small onion, cut into ½-inch pieces
> 2 garlic cloves, crushed with garlic press
> 1 can (28 ounces) reduced-sodium whole tomatoes in juice
> 2 tablespoons tomato paste
> ½ teaspoon salt
> ¼ teaspoon coarsely ground black pepper
> 2 tablespoons chopped fresh basil or parsley

1. In nonreactive 3-quart saucepan, heat oil over medium heat. Add onion and garlic and cook, stirring, until onion is tender, about 5 minutes.

2. Stir in tomatoes with their juice, tomato paste, salt, and pepper; heat to boiling over high heat, stirring to break up tomatoes. Reduce heat to medium and cook, stirring occasionally, until sauce has thickened slightly, about 20 minutes. Stir in basil. Serve over pasta.

Each serving (heaping ½ cup): About 77 calories ■ 2 g protein ■ 8 g carbohydrate ■ 3 g fiber ■ 5 g total fat (1 g saturated) ■ 0 mg cholesterol ■ 255 mg sodium.

Vegetarian

▶ Almost-Instant Rice Salad (14 g fiber)
Instant or quick-cooking brown rice is fine. If you have more time, try brown Texmati or brown Basmati. Have 1 serving.
Prep: 20 minutes ■ Cook: 12 minutes (8 minutes if using leftover rice) ■ Makes 2 servings

⅓ cup brown rice or 1 cup leftover cooked brown rice

salt

2 teaspoons fresh lemon juice

2 teaspoons olive oil

¼ teaspoon ground cumin

pepper

1½ cups canned garbanzo beans or cannellini beans, rinsed and
  drained

⅓ cup crumbled feta cheese

1 to 2 green onions, chopped

2 tablespoons fresh parsley, chopped

½ avocado, chopped

1. Prepare rice according to package directions, using ¼ teaspoon salt.

2. Meanwhile, in small bowl whisk lemon juice, oil, cumin, a pinch of salt, and pepper to taste until blended.

3. In medium bowl, mix beans, feta, green onions, tomato, parsley, and cooked rice; gently stir in avocado.

Each serving: About 491 calories ▪ 18 g protein ▪ 64 g carbohydrate ▪ 14 g fiber ▪ 20 g total fat (6 g saturated) ▪ 22 mg cholesterol ▪ 329 mg sodium.

▌**Avocado and Black Bean Salad** (27 g fiber)

Have 1 serving.

Prep: 20 minutes ▪ Makes 2 servings

1 avocado, pitted and peeled

2 medium plum tomatoes (12 ounces)

2 medium navel oranges

1 can (15 to 19 ounces) black beans, rinsed and drained

⅔ cup no-sodium-added canned whole-kernel corn, drained (or
  defrosted frozen or cooked fresh corn kernels)

1 tablespoon chopped fresh cilantro or parsley

¼ teaspoon salt

1. Cut avocado and tomatoes into bite-size chunks.

2. Cut peel and white pith from oranges; discard. Cut each orange crosswise into ¼-inch-thick slices.

3. In large bowl, combine avocado, tomatoes, orange slices, beans, corn, cilantro, and salt; toss to mix.

Each serving: About 475 calories ▪ 19 g protein ▪ 72 g carbohydrate ▪ 22 g fiber ▪ 16 g total fat (2 g saturated) ▪ 0 mg cholesterol ▪ 346 mg sodium.

Tuscan White Bean Bruschetta with salad (8 g fiber)

Have 2 slices bruschetta with a feta-topped salad: 2 cups mixed greens, 1 cup chopped vegetables (such as tomatoes and mushrooms), 1 tablespoon oil/vinegar dressing, and 2 tablespoons feta.

▶ Tuscan White Bean Bruschetta

Prep: 15 minutes ▪ Grill: 10 minutes ▪ Makes 4 servings

> 1 loaf (8 ounces) Italian bread
> 1 can (15½ to 19 ounces) white kidney beans (cannellini),
>   rinsed and drained
> 1 tablespoon fresh lemon juice
> 1 teaspoon minced fresh sage leaves
> ¼ teaspoon salt
> ⅛ teaspoon coarsely ground black pepper
> 3 tablespoons olive oil
> 3 teaspoons minced fresh parsley leaves
> 2 garlic cloves, each cut in half

1. Prepare grill. Trim ends from bread; reserve for making crumbs or another use. Slice loaf diagonally into eight (½-inch-thick) slices.

2. In medium bowl, with fork, lightly mash beans with lemon juice, sage, salt, pepper, 1 tablespoon oil, and 2 teaspoons parsley.

3. Place bread slices on hot grill rack over medium heat and grill until lightly toasted, 3 to 5 minutes on each side. Rub one side of each toast slice with cut side of garlic. Brush with remaining 2 tablespoons olive oil.

4. Just before serving, top toast slices with bean mixture and sprinkle with remaining parsley.

Tip: To add extra flavor to the beans, use a fruity, full-bodied extra-virgin olive oil.

Each serving (2 slices): About 339 calories ▪ 11 g protein ▪ 45 g carbohydrate ▪ 6 g fiber ▪ 13 g total fat (2 g saturated) ▪ 0 mg cholesterol ▪ 514 mg sodium.

Vegetable pizza with salad (12 g fiber)

Your choices: Make the Whole-Wheat Pita Pizza with Vegetables and have 1 serving. Or heat up a frozen vegetarian pizza. Check labels and have no more than 470 calories. For example: Have two thirds of a 13.2-ounce DiGiorno Spinach Mushroom and Garlic Rising-Crust Pizza or half of Amy's Veggie Combo Pizza. Or pick up the phone and order a vegetarian pizza (e.g., 2½ slices of Domino's Green Pepper, Onions and Mushroom Pizza, or 2 slices of Pizza Hut Hand-Tossed Vegetable Pizza). Since manufacturers frequently reformulate their products, check national chain websites for nutrition information before ordering.

To any of the above, add a side salad: 2 cups mixed greens tossed with ½ teaspoon olive oil, salt and pepper, and lemon juice or vinegar to taste.

▶ Whole-Wheat Pita Pizzas with Vegetables

Prep: 10 minutes ▪ Cook: 25 minutes ▪ Makes 4 servings

1 teaspoon olive oil
1 medium red onion, sliced
2 garlic cloves, crushed with garlic press
¼ teaspoon crushed red pepper
8 ounces broccoli flowerets, cut into 1½-inch pieces
¼ cup water
½ teaspoon salt
1 can (15 to 19 ounces) garbanzo beans, rinsed and drained
1 cup part-skim ricotta cheese
4 (6-inch) whole-wheat pitas, each split horizontally in half
½ cup grated Parmesan cheese
2 medium plum tomatoes (12 ounces), cut into ½-inch chunks

1. Preheat oven to 450°F. In nonstick 12-inch skillet, heat oil over medium-high heat until hot. Add onion and cook, stirring occasionally, until golden, 7 to 10 minutes. Add garlic and crushed red pepper and cook, stirring, 30 seconds. Add broccoli flowerets, water, and ¼ teaspoon salt; heat to boiling. Reduce heat to medium and cook, covered, until broccoli is tender-crisp, about 5 minutes.

2. Meanwhile, in small bowl, with potato masher or fork, mash beans with ricotta and remaining ¼ teaspoon salt until almost smooth.

3. Arrange pita halves on two large cookie sheets. Bake until lightly toasted, about 3 minutes. Spread toasted pitas with bean mixture. Top with broccoli mixture and sprinkle with Parmesan. Bake until heated through, 7 to 10 minutes longer.

4. To serve, sprinkle pitas with tomatoes.

Each pizza: About 469 calories ▪ 27 g protein ▪ 64 g carbohydrate ▪ 10 g fiber ▪ 13 g total fat (6 g saturated) ▪ 29 mg cholesterol ▪ 969 mg sodium.

Calcium Break

Have one of these high-calcium foods every day. American women don't get enough calcium, a mineral critical to strong bones and a healthy heart. Also, research indicates that getting enough calcium may help you lose weight and keep it off. You need 1,000 mg calcium daily up until age fifty. From age fifty-one on, you need 1,200 mg. (These numbers apply to both men and women.) The snacks below are about 100 calories each and provide 300 mg calcium (except the cheese and crackers and the soup which provide 250 mg calcium each). This, in addition to the 300 mg calcium you get courtesy of the dairy serving at each breakfast, ensures 600 mg of calcium daily. You should get another 300 to 400 mg via the calcium sprinkled throughout the rest of the Keep On Losin' plan (in cheese, milk, yogurt, and the smaller amounts in beans and vegetables in the meals). That should be enough for those of you who need 1,000 mg calcium daily. But it doesn't hurt—and will probably help—to take a standard multi as well. Check your multi. It should provide about 100 to 200 mg calcium. Those of you age fifty-one and over need to take a calcium supplement providing 200 to 500 mg calcium daily on top of your multi.

Cheese and crackers: About 45 calories of any whole-grain cracker (e.g., 2 Ak Maks) and 1 slice of reduced-fat Cheddar or American cheese providing about 250 mg—or 25 percent of the DV—of calcium per slice (e.g., Borden's 2% Singles or Cabot 50% Reduced Cheddar).

▶ Chocolate Milk

Mix 1 *heaping teaspoon chocolate syrup* into *1 cup fat-free milk or calcium-enriched rice or soy milk* (check the label for about 90 calories per cup).

▶ Cool Cucumber Soup

Have 1 serving.
Prep: 10 minutes ▪ Makes 4 servings (about 4 cups)

    1 pound cucumbers (2 medium), peeled, seeded, and coarsely
        chopped
    1 container (16 ounces) plain low-fat yogurt
    ½ cup cold water
    1 tablespoon fresh lemon juice
    ¾ teaspoon salt
    ¼ teaspoon coarsely ground black pepper
    1 cup ice cubes
    ¼ cup coarsely chopped fresh mint

In blender, puree cucumbers, yogurt, water, lemon juice, salt and pepper until almost smooth. With motor on and center part of cover removed, add ice cubes, one at a time. Add mint and process 5 seconds to blend.
Each serving: About 88 calories ▪ 7 g protein ▪ 11 g carbohydrate ▪ 1 g fiber ▪ 2 g total fat (1 g saturated) ▪ 7 mg cholesterol ▪ 519 mg sodium.

▶ Flavored Steamer

Heat *1 cup fat-free milk* until hot. Add *1 tablespoon flavored syrup (e.g., Torani) or 2 tablespoons sugar-free flavored syrup*. Note: The tablespoon of regular syrup puts this drink at 120 calories, a little more than the rest, so have this snack no more than three times a week. Sugar-free syrup is calorie-free, so no need to limit it.

▶ Hot Chocolate

Stir *2 teaspoons chocolate syrup* into *1 cup hot fat-free milk or calcium-enriched soy milk*. Or opt for Swiss Miss Sugar-Free Hot Chocolate.

▶ Flavored Yogurt

Stir *1 teaspoon maple syrup* into *⅔ cup plain low-fat yogurt*. Or mix *6 ounces plain low-fat yogurt* (90 to 110 calories, depending on the brand) with *1 teaspoon honey* and *2 tablespoons fresh fruit,* chopped or crushed.

Skim milk: 1 cup

Skim milk latte: 12 ounces. Mix 8 ounces fat-free milk with 2 shots of espresso.

Soy or rice milk, calcium-enriched: Check labels for about 90 calories per cup.

Snacks and Alcohol

Have one of the following 125-calorie foods daily. As often as possible, choose from the "Fruit Snack" category.

FRUIT SNACKS (125 CALORIES EACH)

Apple and cheddar: 1 small apple (about 4 ounces) with a ¾-ounce slice reduced-fat Cheddar.

Berries and honey yogurt: 1 cup halved strawberries or ½ cup blueberries or ¾ cup raspberries dipped in ⅓ cup plain low-fat yogurt mixed with 1 teaspoon honey.

▶ Broiled Brown Sugar Banana

Prep: 5 minutes ■ Broil: 5 minutes ■ Makes 1 serving

> 1 ripe banana, unpeeled
> 2 teaspoons brown sugar
> 1 teaspoon reduced-fat, trans fat–free margarine
> dash cinnamon

1. Preheat broiler. Slit banana lengthwise, being careful not to cut all the way through and leaving 1 inch uncut at ends. (Banana should open, but sides stay connected by the uncut parts of the skin.)

2. In small cup, with fork, blend brown sugar, margarine, and cinnamon until smooth.

3. Place banana cut side up on rack in broiling pan. Spoon brown-sugar mixture into split banana. Place pan in broiler at closest position to heat source. Broil banana until browned, about 5 minutes. Serve banana in skins, with spoon to scoop out fruit.

Each banana: About 136 calories ▪ 1 g protein ▪ 34 g carbohydrate ▪ 3 g fiber ▪ 2 g total fat (0 g saturated) ▪ 0 mg cholesterol ▪ 33 mg sodium.

Dried fruit and nuts: 2 tablespoons dried fruit and scant 2 tablespoons nuts. Dried cranberries, dried plums (prunes), and dried apricots are particularly nutritious.

Fruit: Choose from the following: 1 large banana, 2 large kiwis, 1 heaping cup grapes, 2 cups cantaloupe or honeydew chunks, 2 medium oranges, 2¾ cup strawberry halves, 1½ cups blueberries, 1½ medium apples, or 1 large pear.

Fresh Fruit Salad: 1½ cups fresh fruit salad

▶ Herb-Poached Peaches
Have 1 serving.
Prep: 20 minutes plus chilling ▪ Cook: 35 minutes ▪ Makes 4 servings

> 2 large lemons, plus 1 small lemon, thinly sliced, for garnish
> 2¼ cups water
> ¼ cup sugar
> 1 bay leaf
> 3 thyme sprigs
> 4 firm, ripe peaches (about 1½ pounds)
> 1 tablespoon peach jam

1. Grate peel from 1 lemon and squeeze ¼ cup juice from both lemons.

2. In nonreactive 5-quart Dutch oven or saucepot, combine lemon peel, lemon juice, water, sugar, bay leaf, and 2 thyme sprigs.

3. Peel peaches. As each peach is peeled, immediately immerse in lemon juice mixture to prevent discoloration.

4. Heat peach mixture to boiling over high heat, stirring to dissolve sugar. Reduce heat; cover and simmer until peaches are tender, 5 to 10 minutes. With slotted spoon, transfer peaches to a bowl.

5. Heat poaching liquid to boiling over high heat; cook, uncovered, until liquid is reduced to about 1½ cups, about 15 minutes. Stir in peach jam until dissolved. Pour hot syrup over peaches in bowl. Cool slightly.

6. Cover and refrigerate, turning peaches occasionally, until well chilled, at least 4 hours.

7. To serve, discard bay leaf. Serve peaches with syrup; garnish with lemon slices and remaining thyme sprig.

Each serving: About 131 calories ▪ 1 g protein ▪ 34 g carbohydrate ▪ 3 g fiber ▪ 0 g total fat (0 g saturated) ▪ 0 mg cholesterol ▪ 2 mg sodium.

Juice: Choose from ¾ cup grape juice, 1 cup apple juice, or 1⅛ cups orange juice.

Mini smoothies
▶ Mango-Strawberry Smoothie
Have 1 smoothie.
Prep: 5 minutes ▪ Makes 2 servings (2½ cups)

    1 cup hulled fresh or frozen unsweetened strawberries
    1 cup mango or apricot nectar, chilled
    ½ cup plain low-fat yogurt
    4 ice cubes

In blender, combine strawberries, mango nectar, yogurt, and ice and blend until mixture is smooth and frothy. Pour into 2 tall glasses. Serve with straws, if you like.

Each smoothie: About 130 calories ▪ 4 g protein ▪ 27 g carbohydrate ▪ 2 g fiber ▪ 1 g total fat (1 g saturated) ▪ 4 mg cholesterol ▪ 48 mg sodium.

▶ Frozen Watermelon Slush

Have 1 smoothie.

Prep: 5 minutes ▪ Makes 3 servings (3½ cups)

3 cups cubed seedless watermelon
1 cup frozen strawberries
½ cup lemon sorbet
½ cup pineapple juice, chilled
2 tablespoons fresh lime juice

In blender, combine watermelon, strawberries, sorbet, pineapple juice, and lime juice and blend until mixture is smooth. Pour into 3 glasses. *Each smoothie:* About 123 calories ▪ 2 g protein ▪ 30 g carbohydrate ▪ 2 g fiber ▪ 1 g total fat (0 g saturated) ▪ 0 mg cholesterol ▪ 7 mg sodium.

Peanut butter–stuffed dates. Stuff 3 pitted dates with a total of 1½ teaspoons peanut butter.

SWEET SNACKS (125 CALORIES EACH)

Angel food cake: ⅛ of 9-inch cake with 1 teaspoon chocolate syrup

Chocolate: 0.9 ounces (25 g)

Chocolate-covered peanuts: 0.9 ounces (25 g), 25 (a little under 3 tablespoons)

Cookies: 0.85 ounces (24 g), 2 small (2¼-inch)

Flan or pudding: ⅓ cup

Frozen fruit juice bar: Choose a 125-calorie bar.

Hard candy: 1.1 ounces (31 g)

Ice cream (light) or frozen yogurt: ½ cup (check label for about 110 calories per half cup) topped with 1 teaspoon chocolate syrup

Jelly beans: 1.1 ounces (33 g), (30 small or 12 large)

Malted milk balls: 0.9 ounces (26 g), (about 9 smallish balls)

Mini donuts: 1 ounce, 2 mini donuts or 2 donut holes

SALTY SNACKS (125 CALORIES EACH)
Chips and dip
3 tablespoons sour cream–based dip or 3 tablespoons Black Bean Dip with ½ ounce baked tortilla chips.

▌ Black Bean Dip
Prep: 5 minutes ■ Cook: 5 minutes ■ Makes 11 servings (about 2 cups)

> 4 garlic cloves, peeled
> 1 can (15 to 19 ounces) black beans, rinsed and drained
> 2 tablespoons tomato paste
> 2 tablespoons olive oil
> 5 teaspoons fresh lime juice
> ½ teaspoon ground cumin
> ½ teaspoon ground coriander
> ½ teaspoon salt
> ⅛ teaspoon ground red pepper (cayenne)

1. In 1-quart saucepan, place garlic and enough *water to cover;* heat to boiling over high heat. Reduce heat; cover and simmer 3 minutes. Reserve ¾ cup blanching water. Drain garlic.

2. In blender, combine ½ cup reserved water and garlic; blend until smooth. Add beans, tomato paste, oil, lime juice, cumin, coriander, salt, and ground red pepper. Blend until smooth, adding remaining ¼ cup reserved water if necessary, until mixture reaches dipping consistency.

3. Spoon dip into bowl; cover and refrigerate up to 2 days.

Each 3 tablespoons: About 62 calories ■ 3 g protein ■ 7 g carbohydrate ■ 3 g fiber ■ 3 g total fat (0 g saturated) ■ 0 mg cholesterol ■ 130 mg sodium.

Popcorn: Regular, scant 2 cups, or reduced-fat, 3½ cups

Potato chips: Regular, 0.8 ounce (23 g); or reduced-fat, 1.1 ounces (31 g). Since chip size differs among brands, estimate the amount by looking at the total ounces of the package and doing a little division. Even better: Play it safe by buying small bags, which are usually around 1 ounce.

Pretzels: 1.2 ounces (33 g), about 11 regular ring-shaped pretzels,

Salted nuts: 2½ tablespoons

Spinach snacks: Look for Health is Wealth Spinach Munchees (frozen spinach-filled whole-wheat puffs) or Amy's Spinach Feta Snacks. Check label to confirm calories as manufacturers often reformulate products.

Venison or turkey jerky: 1 ounce (29 g)

Whole-wheat crackers with cream cheese and smoked salmon: About 45 calories of whole-wheat crackers spread with 3 teaspoons reduced-fat cream cheese and 1 ounce smoked salmon

ALCOHOL (125 CALORIES)
Beer: 10 ounces regular or 15 ounces light

Bloody Mary: 5 ounces

Daiquiri: frozen, 2½ ounces

Gin and Tonic: 5 ounces

Hard liquor (gin, vodka, whiskey): 1 jigger (1½ ounces)

Margarita: 2 ounces (small cocktail, not the frozen type)

Martini: 2 ounces

Wine, red or white: 6 ounces

Wine cooler: 8 ounces

BE YOUR OWN NUTRITIONIST

Want to try your hand at designing your own meals? Go for it, using "exchanges," or serving sizes within various food groups as outlined below. Try this only after you've closely followed the Keep On Losin' meals for a few weeks. Those meals teach you about portion size and nutrition balance, making it easier to invent meals and snacks that keep you at 1,500 calories daily.

The beauty of the exchange system is that you don't have to count calories. Instead, you simply count up how many servings of dairy, fats, fruit, protein, snacks, starches, and vegetables you eat. As you become familiar with these portion sizes, you'll be able to quickly size up your meal. For instance, you'll scan your plate and see that the chicken leg is 1 protein serving, the broccoli comes to 2 vegetable servings, and the cup of rice is 2 starch servings. This skill will also come in very handy when you analyze your food diary. You can tally up the serving sizes and see where you're over- or underdoing it.

Follow this approach and you'll stay at about 1,500 calories daily. Your breakfasts, lunches, and dinners will work out like the meals in the Keep On Losin' plan if you use the serving sizes and food groups suggested here. For instance, all the breakfasts on the plan have 1 fruit serving and 1 dairy serving. Most have 2 starches, and all have 1 or 2 fats. In addition to these meals, add on a "Calcium Break" food (page 122) and a 125-calorie treat or snack (page 124).

Size Up Your Meal

Dairy (100 calories per serving)
Have 2 servings per day (1 at breakfast and as a snack)
Examples of 1 serving:
*   1 cup (8 ounces) skim or 1% milk or soy milk
*   6 to 8 ounces plain nonfat, low-fat or artificially sweetened yogurt

Fats (45 calories per serving)
Have 5 servings per day (1 to 2 at every meal)
Examples of 1 serving:
*   1 teaspoon oil, butter, margarine or mayo
*   1 tablespoon salad dressing, cream cheese, or reduced-fat mayo
*   1 slice bacon
*   2 tablespoons reduced-fat cream cheese or salad dressing
*   1 tablespoon nuts

Fruit (60 calories per serving)
Have at least 1 serving per day (at breakfast). Opt for fruit as often as possible for your daily snack.

Examples of 1 serving:

- 1 piece of fruit (e.g. apple, pear)
- 1 cup fruit or 4 ounces juice

Protein (165 calories per serving)
Have 2 servings per day (1 at lunch and dinner)
Examples of 1 serving:

- 3 ounces chicken, fish, lean meat
- 1 cup beans (count also as 2 starches)
- 1 cup tofu
- 2 eggs
- 2 ounces reduced-fat cheese
- ¾ cup 2% cottage cheese or 1 cup 1% cottage cheese
- 3 tablespoons peanut butter (count also as 3 fats)

If you go with the lean protein choices, you are allowed all five of your fat servings. But if you choose a protein with a higher fat content, such as a burger, ribs or chicken with skin, that also includes 2 fat servings. In addition, 2 ounces regular cheese uses up 2 fat servings. So, if you have a grilled cheese sandwich using regular full-fat Cheddar, that uses 2 of your fat servings for that day. But 2 ounces reduced-fat cheese (70 calorie per ounce) doesn't use up any fats. Count 3 tablespoons peanut butter as 1 protein and 3 fats.

Starches (80 calories per serving)
Have 6 servings per day (2 at every meal)
Examples of 1 serving:

- 1 slice bread
- ¼ large bagel
- ½ English muffin
- ½ cup cooked rice, pasta or other grain;
- 80 calories of cereal (check label)
- ½ cup cooked oatmeal
- 4-inch pancake
- ½ large baked potato or sweet potato
- heaping ½ cup cooked potatoes (not fried!)

- half cup cooked corn or peas
- ⅓ cup beans (such as black beans)
- 80-calorie tortilla

Vegetables (25 calories per serving)
Have at least 4 servings per day (1-3 at lunch and dinner)
Examples of 1 serving:
- 2 cups lettuce
- 1 cup chopped raw vegetable
- ½ cup cooked vegetable

HOW TO DESIGN YOUR OWN BREAKFAST

The breakfasts on the Keep On Losin' plan come to an average of 375 calories. A great way to distribute these calories is: 2 starches (160 calories), 1 dairy (100 calories), 1 fruit (60 calories), and 1 fat (45 calories)—allowing 10 calories for wiggle room. That way you ensure a dairy serving—automatically covering about a third of your daily calcium needs—and allow for whole-grain pancakes, breads, cereals, and other breakfast foods.

For instance, if you like bread and cheese for breakfast (a type of breakfast not included in the plan), here's how you'd design it:

2 slices whole-grain bread (2 starches)
1¹/₂ slices low-fat cheese, which according to the label comes to 100 calories (1 dairy)
1 orange (1 fruit)
1 tablespoon almonds (1 fat)

Here's how a pancake breakfast breaks down:

2 buckwheat pancakes (2 starches): If you make them on a nonstick skillet with a little oil spray, no need to use up a fat. But if you use oil or margarine to cook them, then you've used up 1 fat per pancake.
2 teaspoons syrup: Check label; these calories come out of your daily 125-calorie snack.
1 cup berries (1 fruit)
1 cup fat-free milk (1 dairy)

HOW TO DESIGN YOUR OWN LUNCH

The lunches on this plan are about 400 calories each. A balanced way to distribute the calories: 2 starches (160 calories), 1 protein (165 calories); 2 vegetables (50 calories), 1 fat (45 calories). (OK, that comes to 420 calories. But remember: You might have 10 calories from breakfast that you didn't use, and these are just approximates!)

Say you're hankering for a roast beef sandwich. Here's how you'd figure the food groups:

2 slices whole-wheat bread (2 starches)
2 teaspoons reduced-fat mayo (1 fat)
3 ounces lean roast beef (1 protein)
horseradish (so low-calorie it's free!)
tomato slices
On the side: the remaining tomato slices (1 vegetable) and 1/2 cup baby
    carrots (1 vegetable)

Soups are trickier. Here you have to use the nutrition label for help. For instance:

1 cup chicken noodle or chicken and rice soup (label tells you 80 calories
    per cup). Since there's usually not much chicken, count this as 1
    starch
1 slice reduced-fat mozzarella (1/2 protein) melted on 1 slice whole-wheat
    bread (1 starch)
1 large tomato, sliced (2 vegetables) with another slice of reduced-fat
    mozzarella (1/2 protein), drizzled with 1 teaspoon olive oil (1 fat)

HOW TO DESIGN YOUR OWN DINNER

Here is a classic and nutritionally balanced way to design a 500-calorie dinner: 2 starches (160 calories), 1 protein (165 calories), 2 vegetables (50 calories), 2 fats (90 calories). That leaves you 35 calories to play with: perhaps a little bit more rice or a dab more salad dressing or a little more meat.

For instance, here's how it works for a chicken-broccoli stir-fry:

$3/4$ cup chicken (1 protein)
$1^1/_2$ cups broccoli (2 vegetables)
2 teaspoons canola oil for stir-frying (2 fats)
garlic, ginger, soy sauce (all so low-calorie they're free!)
1 cup brown rice (2 starches).

Here's how a fajita dinner breaks down:

2 small tortillas (check label: 80 calories equal 1 starch)
3 ounces flank steak (a lean meat, counts as 1 protein)
1 cup peppers and onions (2 vegetables) sautéed in 1 teaspoon olive oil
     (1 fat)
2 tablespoons reduced-fat sour cream (1 fat)
2 to 3 tablespoons salsa (take it, it's free!)

DESSERT AND SNACKS

The breakfasts, lunches, and dinners outlined above come to 1,275 calories. Bring your day up to 1,500 calories with a 125-calorie snack or dessert (see lists, page 124) and a 100-calorie high-calcium food or beverage (see "Calcium Break," page 122).

5 Burn the Fat

If you don't consider yourself active, yet you've been known to shop, garden, or beach-comb for hours, you're a good candidate for exercise. In other words, *everyone* can do it. Sure, *exercise* can be a scary word if you haven't been getting much, but *obesity* and *heart disease* are even scarier words. Here's the deal: You *can* lose weight without exercising, but it's much harder to do, and you lower your odds of keeping the weight off. Exercise does lots more than burn body fat; it also helps stave off heart disease, cancer, diabetes, osteoporosis, depression, colds and flus, and other conditions. It's just as important as cutting calories, so it's a must on *The Supermarket Diet.*

This chapter will show you just what to do to burn fat and tone your body. You'll be mixing it up with aerobic exercise (like walking), strength training (like weight lifting), and stretching. And just as *The Supermarket Diet* meals don't require fancy or particularly expensive foods, the exercise plan is low budget as well. Here's all you'll need:

- *Good walking shoes or walking sandals*
- *Athletic socks* (to wear with walking shoes)
- *Comfortable walking clothes*
- *Free weights.* These range in price from about $2 for lighter weights to $15 for heavier weights. You should spend some time in a sports shop, feeling the weights to figure out which ones are right for you. Take this book with you and try some of the strength-training exercises at different weights, or simply use the weights at your gym. If you don't belong to a gym, ask for a one-day free trial and sample the weights on that day. Who knows? You may like the gym and join! You'll probably need a pair of lighter weights (maybe 2 pounds) for some exercises and heavier weights (8 pounds or more) for other exercises.

- *Calendar.* It may seem silly to scribble in "walk" on Monday between 7:00 and 8:00 P.M., but it helps. Losing weight is as much about finding time to exercise and go grocery shopping as it is about motivation. It's so easy to fill up the day and leave no time for these key activities. Sure, it's going to mean sacrificing something else—maybe you won't be able to meet your friends for dinner or get the laundry done that night—but you're on a mission: Weight loss must become one of your top priorities. So stay focused, and schedule in the workouts.

The two hardest things about physical activity are getting started and sticking with it long-term. (See Chapter 8, "Staying Slim: The Maintenance Program," for inspiration on sticking with it.) Once you get into it, your body will respond by adapting quickly and revving up for even more. People in their nineties who take up exercise have seen dramatic increases in strength and endurance; so can you.

It might not seem this way to exercise-phobes, but weight loss is a lot easier when you exercise. To lose a pound a week, you have to subtract 500 calories a day. Dropping all 500 calories through diet is pretty depriving; that's an entire meal's worth of calories! But divvy it up between 250 calories of physical activity and 250 calories of food takes the sting out. Plus there's a bonus: Regular exercise suppresses appetite, so you won't be as hungry. Research bears it out time after time: People lose more weight and increase their chances of keeping it off with the combo of healthy eating and regular physical activity.

NO PAIN, BIG GAINS

More good news: You really don't need superstrenuous, painful exercise to lose weight. Countless people have dropped the pounds by just walking. In fact, you burn more fat walking or doing moderately difficult cycling or other moderate activities than you do with very intense exercise that leaves you panting.

Exercise intensity has nothing to do with weight loss. What *did* make a difference in a University of Pittsburgh study: the number of calories burned weekly. Women who burned 2,000 calories a week lost, on average, 19 pounds. But it didn't matter whether they were in the sweaty, vigorous exercising group or the more leisurely exercising group. And women who burned 1,000 calories weekly lost, on average, 15 pounds.

Can You Be Fit and Fat?

If you're one of those overweight people who leaves your skinny friends panting in the dust, your fitness may be as—or more—protective than their thinness. Some studies find that your treadmill test score is much more important than the number on the scale. For instance, studies at the Cooper Institute in Dallas, Texas, showed that avoiding a sedentary lifestyle dramatically cuts the risk of death, no matter what the body weight.

However, other research has found that even if you're fit, if you've got an excess of belly fat—a particular type called "visceral fat"—then you're still at risk. Visceral fat lodges around the organs in the belly area and is linked to heart disease and diabetes. That's in contrast to "subcutaneous" fat, which is right under the skin. A woman who is *not* overweight but has high levels of visceral fat is at higher risk for disease than the woman who is technically overweight, but has little visceral fat (her fat is mostly subcutaneous).

Since you can't tell where your fat is stored—pinching your belly won't tell you—the best advice is to aim for a healthy weight and to stay fit.

GOOD-BYE FAT, HELLO LEAN

As great as walking and other aerobic exercises are, there's something else you need for that real weight-loss edge: strength training. Lifting weights sounds a little tough if you've never done it, but it's actually pretty easy. If you strength-train while losing weight, more of your weight loss will be fat. If you don't strength-train, you lose both muscle and fat. That's because strength training builds your lean muscle tissue. You'll wind up with a more beautifully toned body and a faster metabolism. As you may already know, the more lean tissue you have the higher your rate of metabolism (read: calorie burning). That's because it doesn't take the body much effort to maintain its fat stores, but muscle demands more calories to feed and maintain.

Strength training also helps stave off osteoporosis by increasing bone density. In a twelve-month study at Tufts University, 39 postmenopausal women who had just two days per week of progressive strength training gained muscle mass and an average of 1 percent in hip and spine bone density, increased their strength by 35 to 75 percent and also improved balance. Compare these results to those of a control group who did not strength-train and experienced losses in bone density, strength, and balance. If you're older, strength training helps prevent falls, which translates to fewer fractures.

WHAT'S ENOUGH EXERCISE?

To lose weight, the leading exercise authorities recommend anywhere from a minimum of 30 minutes a day five times a week, to 1 hour daily. Since you bought this book to lose weight, shoot for the higher end: the hour daily. That, in combination with the Boot Camp and Keep On Losin' programs will take weight off most quickly.

Medical Green Light to Exercise

If you've been sedentary, and especially if you're sedentary and over fifty years old, check with your doctor before you start this exercise program. The last thing you need is to pull a tendon and become *really* sedentary or wind up with heart arrhythmias (irregular heart beat) or worse. The doctor should give you a stress electrocardiogram (ECG) and check your blood pressure.

If you've got a chronic disease, such as a heart condition, arthritis, diabetes, or high blood pressure, then consult your doc about what types of physical activity (and how much) are appropriate. Also get a doctor's advice on exercise if you have ever had chest pain (especially chest pain that is brought on by exertion), loss of balance (especially loss of balance leading to a fall), dizziness, or loss of consciousness.

No matter what physical condition you're in, the physical activity readiness questionnaire (PAR-Q) on page 275 will help you determine if you should check with your doctor before you start.

Timing Meals and Workouts

Your stomach's growling on your way to the gym. Should you eat something before exercising? Yes, a little something, because you want to make it through your workout without hunger or lightheadedness. However, you don't want to eat too much before exercising; it'll weigh you down, diminishing performance, and could give you belly cramps. Below are three basic rules of thumb. Since everyone's digestion rate is different, experiment, and modify the amount you eat accordingly.

▶ Include at least one starch serving in the meal before exercise. A starch serving is: 1 slice of bread, $1/3$ cup cooked rice, $1/2$ cup cooked pasta or potatoes, 80 calories of crackers or any other starchy food. Starch supplies your muscles with glycogen, the body's storage form of sugar. When you start exercising, that glycogen gets converted to quick energy.

▶ Give food time to digest. After a large meal, allow 3 to 4 hours before exercising, 2 to 3 hours following a smaller meal, and less than an hour after a snack. So, if you need a little boost shortly before your workout, have a banana, or half a sweetened yogurt, or a tablespoon of nuts and a small apple.

▶ There's no "magic" time to exercise. The best time to exercise is when you have the time. Aim for 35 to 40 minutes of aerobic exercise (preceded by a warm-up and followed by a cooldown) three to five days a week. If you're trying to lose weight, do this five or more days a week.

The hour daily recommendation comes from the National Academy of Sciences, a highly respected organization that also determines the recommended daily requirements of vitamins and minerals. You need that hour to make a dent in body fat, lower blood pressure, and help prevent a host of diseases. But you don't have to get it all at once. Accumulate that hour in 15-minute intervals or even shorter spurts (such as the 2-minute climb up the stairs to your office).

As for strength training, it should be part of your exercise routine for a minimum of two days a week; three days a week is ideal.

Walking/Aerobics Program

Aerobic exercise is the type that gets you huffing and puffing (but not *too* much!), forcing your body to burn extra calories. A brisk walk is aerobic, so is time spent swimming laps or on a treadmill, elliptical exerciser, stair-stepper, bicycle, rowing machine, or any other of the many ways we can get our heart rates up and burn some fat. Studies show not only that are you burning more calories while working out but also that you continue to burn calories at a jacked-up rate even hours later.

Build from your current level of aerobic activity. If you are sedentary, then follow the Walking Program for Beginners. If you're getting some sort of aerobic exercise twice a week, say walking for 40 minutes and taking a 45-minute aerobics class, your mission is to build up to more days per week. Ditto for more rigorous exercisers: Add a little more time to your workouts, or work out more days of the week.

Eventually, even if it takes six months, you can build up to about an hour of aerobic activity nearly every day. Sounds like a lot? Remember: The more you exercise, the more you can eat. That second serving of mashed potatoes won't have the dire consequences it had when you were sedentary. Not that you can gorge yourself, but you can relax a little. The occasional food slip-ups will be countered by your workouts.

Ready or not, open your calendars and PDAs and schedule in aerobic exercise at least three days this week. Those who have been sedentary should follow the Walking Program for Beginners on the next page. Others can follow this schedule:

WEEK 1: At least three days this week, walk (or do another aerobic activity) at least 30 minutes. Warm up with a slow, 5-minute walk and end with a slow 5-minute walk to cool down.

WEEK 2: Four days this week, walk (or do another aerobic activity) at least 40 minutes. Warm up with a slow, 5-minute walk and end with a slow 5-minute walk to cool down.

WEEK 3 and BEYOND: Walk (or do another aerobic activity) at least an hour, 6 days a week. Warm up with a slow, 5-minute walk and end with a slow 5-minute walk to cool down.

WALKING PROGRAM FOR BEGINNERS

If you've been sedentary, or have a chronic condition, and/are over age fifty, play it safe and stick with the following beginners' walking program, which was adapted, with permission, from the National Heart, Lung and Blood Institute. Follow the guidelines in the following chart to determine the amount of walking: In weeks one and two, take at least three walks a week; in week three, increase your exercise to take at least four walks; then in weeks four and beyond, take at least five walks a week.

WEEK 1 (at least 3 walks)

Warm-up	Walk slowly 5 minutes
Activity	Walk briskly 5 minutes
Cool-down	Walk slowly 5 minutes
Total Time	15 minutes

WEEK 2 (at least 3 walks)

Warm-up	Walk slowly 5 minutes
Activity	Walk briskly 7 minutes
Cool-down	Walk slowly 5 minutes
Total Time	17 minutes

WEEK 3 (at least 4 walks)

Warm-up	Walk slowly 5 minutes
Activity	Walk briskly 9 minutes
Cool-down	Walk slowly 5 minutes
Total Time	19 minutes

WEEK 4 (at least 5 walks)

Warm-up	Walk slowly 5 minutes
Activity	Walk briskly 11 minutes
Cool-down	Walk slowly 5 minutes
Total Time	21 minutes

WEEK 5 (at least 5 walks)

Warm-up	Walk slowly 5 minutes
Activity	Walk briskly 13 minutes
Cool-down	Walk slowly 5 minutes
Total Time	23 minutes

WEEK 6 (at least 5 walks)

Warm-up	Walk slowly 5 minutes
Activity	Walk briskly 15 minutes
Cool-down	Walk slowly 5 minutes
Total Time	25 minutes

WEEK 7 (at least 5 walks)

Warm-up	Walk slowly 5 minutes
Activity	Walk briskly 18 minutes
Cool-down	Walk slowly 5 minutes
Total Time	28 minutes

WEEK 8 (at least 5 walks)

Warm-up	Walk slowly 5 minutes
Activity	Walk briskly 20 minutes
Cool-down	Walk slowly 5 minutes
Total Time	30 minutes

WEEK 9 (at least 5 walks)

Warm-up	Walk slowly 5 minutes
Activity	Walk briskly 23 minutes
Cool-down	Walk slowly 5 minutes
Total Time	33 minutes

WEEK 10 (at least 5 walks)

Warm-up	Walk slowly 5 minutes
Activity	Walk briskly 26 minutes
Cool-down	Walk slowly 5 minutes
Total Time	36 minutes

WEEK 11 (at least 5 walks)

Warm-up	Walk slowly 5 minutes
Activity	Walk briskly 28 minutes
Cool-down	Walk slowly 5 minutes
Total Time	38 minutes

WEEK 12 AND BEYOND (at least 5 walks each week)

Warm-up	Walk slowly 5 minutes
Activity	Walk briskly 30 minutes
Cool-down	Walk slowly 5 minutes
Total Time	40 minutes

Pedometer Power

Curious about how many miles a day you walk? A pedometer can tell you—and it can also motivate you to keep beating your record. A mile is about 2,000 footsteps. Women who accumulate 10,000 steps per day are more likely to be in the normal body-weight range. Those who are overweight or obese tend to walk less, according to a University of Tennessee study. And wearing a pedometer motivates people to walk those 10,000 steps. In that study, 106 sedentary workers strapped on pedometers, starting out at an average of 7,000 daily steps. Four weeks later, they averaged 10,480 daily steps and lost weight, lost inches off their waists, and lowered resting heart rates (meaning improved fitness).

Pedometers are most accurate when you walk at least 3 miles an hour. If you walk more slowly, get the more sensitive piezoelectric pedometers, also called *accelerometers*.

Strength Training

I hope you're sold on the beautiful body-sculpting—and bone-preserving—power of strength training. Even if you're not convinced, give it a try and see for yourself. If you belong to a gym, spring for at least one session with a personal trainer who can set you up with a safe routine. Track your progress over the weeks and months with a measuring tape at your waist, hips, thighs, and upper arms.

Your strength-training rules:

- *5–10 minute warm-up.* Before you hit the weights, *always* warm up your muscles by walking or getting on a treadmill, bike, elliptical exerciser, rowing machine, or any other available aerobic equipment. Five or ten minutes is enough to send more blood to your muscles, prepping them to respond better to lifting weights and helping to prevent injury.

SuperTip ➤ Strength-Training Guides

You want your muscles toned but not sore. To strength-train safely, either enlist a personal trainer or get a reputable manual. The *Strong Women* series by Tuft University's Miriam Nelson, Ph.D., and coauthors offers safe and effective strength-training workouts based on research. The series includes *Strong Women Stay Young* (New York: Bantam Books, 2000), *Strong Women, Strong Bones* (New York: Putnam, 2000), and *Strong Women and Men Beat Arthritis* (New York: Putnam, 2002).

Also, the Centers for Disease Control has a wonderful (and free!) program on its website called "Strength Training for Older Adults." This program, also based on Miriam Nelson's research, is not just for older people but works for people of any age. The link: go to www.cdc.gov and search for "strength training."

Stretch to Counter Sore Muscles

After exercising, whether aerobics or strength training, you need to stretch the muscles you've just used. During your workout, your muscles contract thousands of times and become prone to contracting powerfully—and shortening—*after* the workout. This causes muscle soreness. But by gently stretching after exercising, you relax and lengthen the muscle fibers. This doesn't always prevent soreness, but it helps.

Gradually, carefully, stretch arm and leg muscles, going into the stretch slowly, and hold for 30 to 60 seconds. If you like, repeat the stretch after a 1-minute rest. Don't bounce, as bouncing causes the muscle to contract again.

- *Train every other day.* Do the exercises three times a week, leaving one day of rest in between workouts. This allows muscles to rest and repair between sessions. For instance, do them Monday, Wednesday, and Friday, or Tuesday, Thursday, and Saturday.
- *Start gradually.* Even if you feel that the weight is too light, better that than a weight that is too heavy and injures you. Get used to the motion with a light weight and gradually increase to a heavier one. And remember: What feels too light during the first five repetitions gets a lot heavier by the twelfth!
- *Challenge yourself.* Over the course of your weight loss, challenge yourself by gradually increasing the number of repetitions (reps) and perhaps introduce heavier weights. (See "Working at the Right Intensity," opposite.)
- *Stretch.* Finish off each strength-training session with stretching exercises.

Working at the Right Intensity— Judging Your Effort

When exercising, it is important to find the right balance between being careful to prevent injury and always progressing to increase strength. This easy-to-use scale will help you find the right intensity for your workout.

Exercise Intensity Indicator*
  Ask yourself these questions after each exercise:

1. Were you able to complete two sets of ten repetitions in good form? (You should complete each repetition in proper form, using a "2-up, pause, 4-down" count.)
No: Reduce the weight so you can lift ten times in good form; then repeat for a second set.
Yes: Please continue to question 2.

2. After completing ten repetitions, do you need to rest because the weight is too heavy to complete more repetitions in good form?
Yes: You are working at the right intensity and should not increase the weight.
No: Please continue to questions 3 and 4 to determine how to safely increase the intensity of your workout.

3. Could you have done a few more repetitions in good form without a break?
Yes: You may feel that you can do only a few more repetitions, not the entire next set of ten without a break. At your next workout, do the first set of repetitions with the weight you have been using, then do the second set with a slightly heavier weight. For example, if you're currently using 2-pound dumbbells, use 3-pound dumbbells for your second set.

4. Could you have done all twenty repetitions at one time, without a break?
Yes: Use heavier dumbbells for both sets of repetitions the next time you work out. If you are using adjustable ankle weights, you will be able to increase intensity when you're ready by adding $1/2$- or 1-pound weights to each leg.

---

*Courtesy of the Division of Nutrition and Physical Activity, National Center for Chronic Disease Prevention and Health Promotion, Centers for Disease Control.

Part Two
Become a Savvy Shopper

6 Label Literacy: Don't Be Duped!

A client walked into my office, bursting with excitement over her amazing find: A big muffin for just 180 calories! "It's so good, I've been eating one each morning for the last three days," she reported. She handed me the label. She was right. It said "Calories: 180." But, as I sadly pointed out to her, the line above read: "Serving Size: 2 oz. Servings per Package: 4." We multiplied 180 by 4, and to her horror and chagrin, she'd been eating a 720-calorie muffin! Then we weighed it, and it was a good 2 ounces over the stated 8-ounce weight, so make that a 900-calorie muffin. There went more than half her calories for the day.

Finish this chapter, and you won't be unwittingly eating 900-calorie muffins! You'll learn how to read labels and really understand what the numbers mean. I'll also point out ways some food manufacturers try to trick you into believing their product is healthier than it is. You'll soon be a whiz at comparing labels. That ultra-rich, super-premium ice cream bar at 290 calories and 14 g saturated fat? No way. That's just shy of your saturated-fat maximum (15 grams) for the *entire day!* Instead, toss into your cart Starbucks Frappuccino bars or Skinny Cow ice cream sandwiches at 120 to 140 calories and just 1 g of saturated fat. Your label comparisons will also fill your cart with lower-sodium foods, cutting back on bloating and helping reduce blood pressure.

In the next chapter, you'll put your skills to work as you go down the supermarket aisles and learn how to quickly size up a decent cereal or frozen dinner and use the label to choose the best of the rest of your staple items.

Ready to conquer the label? Let's use the "Mac & Cheese" food label as an example. It looks just like any other food label; by law labels have to conform to a standard format.

Quick Guide to the "Nutrition Facts" Food Label

Here is a nutrition facts label for "Mac & Cheese."

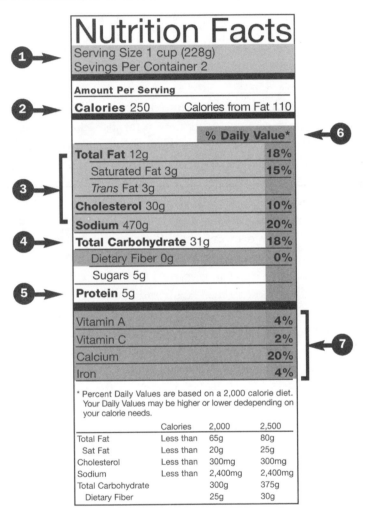

The numbers next to the label correspond to the key on the following page.

1. Serving size. Watch it! Two servings per package, so for this product, the info applies to just half the package.

2. Check calories: Put calories in perspective. Most meals on *The Supermarket Diet* are 400 to 500 calories, snacks 100 to 200.

3. Watch the risky fats: On a 1,500-calorie weight-loss plan, limit *daily* saturated fat to 15 g and trans fats to 1.6 g. In addition, limit cholesterol to 300 mg and sodium to 2,300 mg.

4. Carb watch: Women should aim for 25 g or more of dietary fiber daily, men 38 g. (Dietary fiber is often referred to as fiber, as we do throughout *The Supermarket Diet*.) Naturally occurring sugar in dairy and fruit is OK, but limit added sugar intake as explained in this chapter.

5. Protein: Daily protein should be about 60 g on a 1,200-calorie plan, 75 g on a 1,500-calorie plan, and 90 g on 1,800 calories per day.

6. % DV: Remember, these are very rough guidelines based on consuming 2,000 calories a day—much more than you can afford if you want to lose weight. Daily values for your calorie level on *The Supermarket Diet* are provided on page 160.

7. % DV of vitamins and minerals: This is a good way to compare relative levels of important nutrients, like calcium, among different products. But as explained later in this chapter, overly high levels of some vitamins and minerals are not always desirable.

How to Read and Interpret the "Nutrition Facts" Food Label

SERVING SIZE

Get this wrong and you can wind up in mega-calorie overdose, to say nothing of overdoing saturated fat and other unhealthy components. Check out the labels below, which appear on two brands of flavored rice. Can you figure out which one is higher in calories? In sodium?

At first glance, Brand B seems to save you both calories and sodium. But look closely, and you'll notice the difference in serving size, which makes it very difficult to compare the two. It works out that *per ounce,* Brand A has 95 calories and 495 mg sodium. The Brand B version, *per*

COMPARE THE LABELS		
	Brand A Spanish Rice	**Brand B Spanish Rice**
Serving size	2 ounces	1.5 ounces
Calories	190	140
Sodium	990 mg	570 mg

ounce, has 93 calories and 378 mg sodium. Here's how you figure: Using a calculator, divide the calories by the ounces to get the calories per ounce. For instance, for Brand A, it's 190 divided by 2, which equals 95 calories per ounce. For Brand B brand, it's 140 divided by 1.5, which equals 93 calories per ounce. Do the same for the sodium. Virtually the same calories, but Brand B is easier on sodium. (As you'll read in the next chapter, you're better off making your own flavored rice and saving even more sodium—and dollars!)

CALORIES

On the Keep On Losin' plan, lunches are 400 calories; dinners, 500 calories. On the Stay Slim Maintenance plan you get 500 calories for lunch and 550 to 600 for dinner. Keep those numbers in mind when you shop for or plan a meal. Say you're on the Keep On Losin' plan. You pick up a can of chili for lunch. It's 200 calories per cup, so you can have a cup and a half for 300 calories, then split the remaining 100 calories between corn bread and salad. Or, maybe you have a hankering for Lean Cuisine's Chicken Fettucini, which is just 280 calories, way too little for dinner. Use your label-reading skills to build up calories with extra frozen broccoli, maybe a little grated Parmesan, and fruit for dessert. For snacks, stick to about 125 calories on the Keep On Losin' plan and up to 200 calories on the Maintenance program.

TOTAL FAT

The National Academy of Sciences guidelines for fat consumption are 20 to 35 percent of your total daily calories, which is a wide range, meaning nothing to most people. Much more important than the total fat is the amount of saturated and trans fat in a food. Here's what you need to know about these fats:

Saturated Fat

In excess, sat fat raises blood cholesterol, increasing the risk of heart disease and stroke. It's found naturally in foods, especially concentrated in fatty animal-based foods, such as butter and chicken skin, and in some oils, such as palm and coconut. Even "good" oils like olive and canola oil have a little saturated fat, so you can't avoid it entirely.

A heart-healthy diet should have less than 10 percent of total calories from saturated fat, which is a maximum of 12 g saturated fat daily on the 1,200-calorie Boot Camp plan; 15 g saturated fat on the 1,500-calorie Keep On Losin' plan; and 18 g saturated fat on the Stay Slim Maintenance plan. Look at the bottom of the Mac & Cheese label and remember this part of the label is the same on all packaged foods: the recommended saturated fat maximums of 20 g and 25 g daily are higher than your maximum because the label refers to a 2,000-calorie and 2,500-calorie diet, respectively.

Don't worry, daily allowances are all worked out for you on *The Supermarket Diet* food plans so you don't have to do any daily-allowance calculations. So ignore the saturated-fat recommendations at the bottom of the food label. Instead, zero in on the actual grams of saturated fat in a serving of the food, which is posted toward the top of the label.

Trans Fat

Even worse than saturated fat, trans fat not only raises LDL ("bad cholesterol") but lowers HDL ("good cholesterol"). It's formed by a process called *hydrogenation*, which turns oils into semisolids such as margarine and shortening. You'll notice these oils on the ingredient list as *partially hydrogenated oil* or *shortening* and reflected in the trans fat total in the Nutrition Facts. Try to keep your trans fat intake as low as possible.

CHOLESTEROL AND SODIUM

Cholesterol is a fatlike substance made by the body and taken in through diet. Cholesterol found in food isn't as potent a blood cholesterol–raiser as saturated or trans fat. However, for cholesterol-sensitive people, exces-

Attention Shoppers ➤ Trouncing Trans

After years of badgering by consumer groups, the Food and Drug Administration now requires food manufacturers to post the trans fat content of foods on the food label. But a food with "hydrogenated" or "partially hydrogenated" oil or "shortening"—all sources of trans fat— in the ingredient list may *still* legally claim to have 0 g trans fat. Why? Here's the catch: If a food contains less than half a gram (under 0.5 g) of trans fat, manufacturers can list it as "0." Now half a gram seems like a negligible amount, but some scientists are recommending limiting trans fat to 1 percent of total calories. That's just 1.6 g trans fat on a 1,500-calorie diet like the Keep On Losin' plan; just 2 g on the 1,800-calorie Stay Slim Maintenance plan. At these low limits, those 0.49 g or 0.3 g trans add up quickly: A few cookies, a few teaspoons of margarine are all it takes to exceed your trans fat limit, even though the labels on these foods say "0 trans fat."

It's estimated that the average daily intake of trans fat for adults is about 5.8 grams, or 2.6 percent of calories per day. Now that manufacturers are required to report trans fat, they are trying to remove this fat from their products, so you should have more trans fat–free foods to choose from. You can ensure that your own trans fat numbers are down by comparing labels and following these tips:

▶ Use canola or olive oil when possible.
▶ Limit—or avoid (if possible)—processed foods made with "partially hydrogenated" oils, or with oils high in saturated fat (palm, palm kernel, coconut), and butter.
▶ Use "0 trans" or "trans fat–free" margarine.

sive dietary cholesterol will do damage. The recommended daily limit is 300 mg for the general population, 200 mg for those with high blood cholesterol. Cholesterol is found only in foods of animal origin, so a vegetable oil, while high in fat, would never have cholesterol. (See "Don't Be Duped by Label Gimmicks," page 161)

Sodium can contribute to heart disease by raising blood pressure.

While some individuals tend to be more sodium-sensitive than others, on average, the higher the sodium or salt intake, the higher a person's blood pressure. The latest government recommendation is to have no more than 2,300 mg daily, which amounts to a little less than 1 teaspoon; the recommendation preempts the current information on the Nutrition Facts label, which suggests 2,400 mg as the daily maximum of salt intake. Sounds like a lot until you start picking up cans of soup with 900 mg per cup, or frozen dinners with more than 1,000 mg.

TOTAL CARBOHYDRATES

Despite the bashing they've received at the hand of Atkins and other low-carb diets, carbohydrates—well, the *right kind* of carbohydrates—are actually mainstays of a balanced weight-loss and maintenance plan. Choose breads, crackers, cereals, and even frozen dinners with ingredient lists that lead off with "good" carbs. These include fruits, vegetables, and whole grains such as whole wheat, oats, and whole rye (for more on whole grains see "How to Spot the Whole Grain," page 164). Avoid brands that lead off with the less healthy carbs such as sweeteners and white flour. A rule of thumb for meals: Allow about 45 g of carbs total from starchy foods (such as bread, potatoes, and rice) and from vegetables. You can add a fruit to that, for an additional 15 g.

Total carbohydrates have three components: starch, sugar, and dietary fiber. Dietary fiber and sugar are broken out on the label, and the remaining starch is the amount left over, which can be figured out easily. For instance, a slice of bread has 15 g total carbohydrate, 2 g dietary fiber, and 2 g sugar, leaving 11 g starch. The word *starch* conjures up white bread and mashed potatoes and other foods that dieters have grown to fear, but it's actually an important part of a balanced diet. Remember, good carbs, like oatmeal and whole-wheat pasta, are made up primarily of starch.

There is no daily value for sugar, but the less sugar the better. You don't have to worry about the naturally occurring sugar in milk and yogurt and fruit as long as you're having about three dairy servings and three fruits daily. But you need to limit *added* sugar from sweeteners. Added sugar comes from sugar, high fructose corn syrup, dextrose, fruit juice concentrate, honey, maple syrup, and other sweeteners. Ideally, you

Back in 1966, the average American ate about 113 pounds of sugar per year. As outrageous as that sounds, it crept up to 124 pounds in 1986, then an unbelievable 141.5 pounds in 2003 (the latest stats as of press time). That's 321 cups of sugar, or nearly a cup a day—a whopping 774 calories. And that's *added* sugar (white sugar, high fructose corn syrup, honey, etc.) on top of the sugar found naturally in fruit and dairy products.

In moderation—a little candy a day, or a medium-size cookie, or a few teaspoons of sugar or honey in your tea—sugar isn't bad for you. But mega-amounts are dangerous. A high-sugar diet may raise levels of triglycerides, a blood fat connected with heart disease, and it may increase the risk of diabetes. Foods high in sugar are rarely nutritious, so you displace healthful calories from chicken, milk, vegetables, and the like for nutritionally empty cookies, candy, and other sweets. Or, if you add those foods on top of a healthy diet, you're still in trouble, because of the excess calories. If you see any of these words on the ingredient list, they mean *added sugar:* brown sugar, corn sweetener, corn syrup, dextrose, fructose, fruit juice concentrates, glucose, high-fructose corn syrup, honey, invert sugar, lactose, maltose, malt syrup, molasses, raw sugar, sucrose, sugar, syrup.

should have no more than 24 g added sugar a day (equivalent to 6 teaspoons) on the 1,500-calorie Keep On Losin' plan and no more than 40 g (equivalent to 10 teaspoons) on the 1,800-calorie Maintenance plan. Just one 12-ounce can of soda has 33 g sugar!

Remember, as discussed on page 59, dietary fiber is a strong ally for anyone trying to lose weight. Try to get at least 25 g daily of this slimming disease fighter.

PROTEIN

Protein is a great weight-loss friend; it helps keep you feeling full for hours after eating. However, too much protein is unhealthy; it can stress the kidneys, and if it comes from fatty meats it's also dousing you with saturated fat. (In general, Americans consume too much protein.) On a 1,500-calorie plan, 75 g protein is a healthy amount; about 90 g is OK on an 1,800-calorie plan. Aim for 20 to 25 g protein per meal. A little more or less is fine.

Beef, chicken, fish, pork, lamb, and other meats and tofu and other soy products are the richest sources of protein. Beans (black, pinto, lentils, etc.), cheese, milk, and yogurt are the next highest. Then there is a little protein in grain, bread, and other starches and in vegetables. Ideally, your plate should look like this: half the plate filled with vegetables or fruits, a quarter with starches, and just another quarter for protein-rich foods (and a little fat).

% DAILY VALUE

The Daily Value (DV) is a rough approximation of nutrients people on 2,000- or 2,500-calorie-per-day diets should be consuming. So, the % DV numbers on the label for fat, saturated fat, and total carbohydrates don't apply to any of the lower-calorie plans on *The Supermarket Diet*. Instead, use the numbers in the chart on page 160 as your guide. Remember, a little more or less total fat and a little more or less total carbohydrate is fine, but try to stay within the saturated-fat and fiber recommendations. This chart not only covers the bottom of the food label but offers guidelines on a few other nutrients.

VITAMINS AND MINERALS

The vitamin and mineral standards recommended today by the Food and Drug Administration (FDA) were inherited from decades-old research, which in many cases is off the mark from current recommendations. (The FDA is working on changing this.) In general, the higher the vitamins and minerals in unfortified foods the better. Unfortified foods don't have added vitamins or minerals; the nutrients are found naturally in the foods. For instance, the vitamins A and C in a frozen vegetable-topped pizza come from the tomato, green pepper, and other vegetables. The calcium in the pizza comes from the cheese. (The calcium levels of foods are worth noting. Women typically are deficient in this mineral, which is so critical for strong bones and a healthy heart and seems to play

RECOMMENDED DAILY INTAKES

Download this chart. Go to www. goodhousekeeping. com	Keep On Losin' 1,500 daily calories	Stay Slim Maintenance 1,800 daily calories
Calories	400 to 500 per meal, 125 snack	400 to 600 per meal, up to 200 per snack
Fat	50 g per day	60 g per day
Saturated Fat	15 g per day max.	18 g per day max.
Trans Fat	1.6 g per day max.	2 g per day max.
Cholesterol	300 mg per day max.	300 mg per day max.
Sodium	2,300 mg per day max.	2,300 mg per day max.
Total Carbohydrates	about 190 g per day	225 to 250 g per day
Dietary Fiber	at least 25 g per day	at least 25 g per day
Sugars*	24 g per day max. of *added sugar*	40 g per day max. of *added sugar*
Protein	about 75 g per day	about 90 g per day

*Check the ingredient list for sugar, high-fructose corn syrup, dextrose, or other added sugars. The 12.5 g sugar listed on the label for 1 cup fat-free milk is not added sugar, it's naturally occurring sugar, so it doesn't count toward your daily maximum. But the 12 g sugar in a serving of Keebler Grasshopper cookies? That's added sugar!

a role in weight loss—more on this in chapter 8). But high levels of vitamins and minerals added to fortified foods like cereals and juices can drive up your daily intake to harmful high levels. For instance, after age fifty a woman needs just 8 mg iron daily. If a cereal has 100 % of the DV because of fortification, that's 18 mg. Then there's the iron in her multivitamin, plus the naturally occurring iron in foods. You see how easy it is to get too much. While too little iron causes debilitating anemia, too much of this mineral puts you at risk for heart disease.

How to Interpret Other Packaging Info

INGREDIENT LIST

While the Nutrition Facts panel can tell you a lot about a food, you need to check the ingredient list to see what you're really eating. Ingredients will tell you if you're eating a whole grain or what type of oil is in a salad dressing. The nutrition facts panel doesn't give you that information.

Here's a classically deceptive phrase that frequently appears on bread packages: "wheat bread." Sounds wholesome, doesn't it? You probably think you're getting whole-wheat bread along with its beneficial fiber. But look at the ingredient list, and you'll usually find a disappointing white-flour product that may even have a little caramel coloring thrown in to make it look closer to nature. The first ingredient is probably enriched flour, which means white flour. A glance at the dietary fiber reveals a measly 1 g (sometimes 0.5 g) fiber per slice. Its whole-wheat counterpart, with whole-wheat flour as the first ingredient, would have at least 2 g fiber. So remember, *wheat* usually refers to white flour, but *whole wheat* is the whole grain.

By law, ingredient lists must be ordered by weight. The heaviest ingredient goes first, followed by the next heaviest, and so on. You know you're in trouble when sugar is the first ingredient in cereal (yes, some kids' cereals are *that* sugary) or when bad fats like "partially hydrogenated soybean and cottonseed oils" are ranked as high as the third ingredient in a can of fatty biscuit dough.

You'll get plenty of chances to compare both ingredients and nutrition facts panels in the next chapter.

DON'T BE DUPED BY LABEL GIMMICKS

Beware of these common phrases found on many food packages:

* *Cholesterol Free* or *No cholesterol.* Is that peanut butter or canola oil with "No cholesterol!" splashed across the label better for you than products without that claim? Nope. Turn to the Nutrition Facts

panel and you'll see that no brand of peanut butter or vegetable oil has cholesterol and never did! Only foods of animal origin harbor cholesterol. But manufacturers are hoping you don't know that.

- *Light.* This word can be used to describe fat content, taste, or color, and it's not always crystal clear which it is. If the manufacturer is describing the fat content as "light," the product has at least 50 percent less fat than the original. The manufacturer must also state the fat percentage on the label, as in "50% less fat than our regular cheese." So, light cream cheese is certainly less fatty than regular, but at 35 calories a tablespoon, you still have to watch it. However "light" olive oil—used here to describe the oil's color—is just as caloric as regular but has been processed to remove any distinctive flavor. Or a muffin mix can say "light and fluffy" as a way to describe its texture or consistency. So don't get tricked into thinking that the word *light* necessarily means that you are getting a healthier product! Remember: Unless the label states that the calories, fat, or sodium have been reduced by a percentage from the original product, you're not getting a health benefit.

- *Low fat* or *Fat free.* By law, these products have to be lower in fat than the original or virtually fat free. But check calories; they might be loaded with those! Lots of people have become fat eating too many fat-free cookies and cakes, foods full of starch and sugar . . . and calories!

- *Low sodium* or *Light in sodium.* That means sodium was cut by at least half over the original product. But when you've got a super-high–sodium food like soy sauce or some soups, you might still wind up with a relatively high-sodium product. You can eat these foods, but make sure to factor their sodium level into your daily intake.

- *Sugar-free, No added sugars, Without added sugars.* Yup, that sugar-free chocolate might not have a speck of sugar, but it's still got plenty of fat—and calories. Always turn the package around and find out how many calories and grams of saturated fat you're getting.

- *Sweetened with fruit juice, Fruit juice sweetener,* or *Fruit juice concentrate.* These sweeteners are made by boiling down juice—usually grape juice—into a sticky sweetener. Although they offer a little potassium, these sweeteners are not at all nutritious. Consider them just like sugar.

WHY LOOK FOR WHOLE GRAINS?

Whole-grain eaters are thinner than people who eat few whole grain foods and more processed white flour, according to research at Harvard University and elsewhere. For instance, the Harvard study tracked 74,091 women for ten years and found that women eating the most whole grains weighed less than those who ate the fewest. (Those eating the most whole grain ate 1.62 servings per 1,000 calories. That works out to three servings of whole grain per day on an 1,800-calorie diet. The lowest consumers ate virtually no whole grains.) Also, over the ten-year span, women who ate the most whole grains and other sources of dietary fiber gained less weight than those who ate the least. This wasn't because of a difference in calorie intake, exercise, fruit and vegetable intake, or any other dietary difference. Researchers speculate that the whole grains may beneficially influence hormonal controls of weight, such as reducing insulin, which may decrease fat storage. In other studies, eating more whole grains is linked to a reduced risk of heart disease, diabetes, and certain types of cancer.

Fiber is credited with much of the health benefits of whole grains (see "Slim Down with Fiber," page 59, for more details). That fiber is housed in the bran layer of some grains. When whole wheat is processed to create white flour, that bran layer is removed. That doesn't eliminate just the fiber but also the disease-fighting antioxidants in bran. Also chucked out is the wheat germ, a rich source of E and B vitamins. What's left is the endosperm, the starchy part, which isn't particularly rich in vitamins or minerals. That's why most of the white flour in the U.S. is "enriched"—injected with B vitamins and iron.

Oats and barley are different; they have a type of fiber (beta-glucan) that runs throughout the entire kernel, so even if the outside is removed, you still get fiber. So "pearled" barley, with the outside tough layer removed, is still a good source of fiber.

The latest government recommendations: At least half of your grains should be whole-grain. *The Supermarket Diet* recommendation: 90 to 100 percent whole grains! To cash in on the weight-loss and health benefits of whole grains, first figure out whether you're buying a whole-grain–rich food. It's not always easy to tell. Here are your clues:

How to Spot the Whole Grain in the Ingredients List

It's a whole grain if it's called:

- [ ] Brown rice
- [ ] Buckwheat
- [ ] Bulgur or cracked wheat
- [ ] Millet
- [ ] Quinoa
- [ ] Sorghum
- [ ] Triticale wheat berries
- [ ] Whole-grain barley (Pearled barley is also OK, since it's such a good source of fiber.)
- [ ] Whole-grain corn
- [ ] Whole oats or oatmeal
- [ ] Wild rice
- [ ] Whole rye
- [ ] Whole spelt
- [ ] Whole wheat

It's not a whole grain if it's called:

- [ ] Corn flour
- [ ] Cornmeal
- [ ] Degerminated cornmeal
- [ ] Enriched flour
- [ ] Multigrain (This simply means it's composed of various grains, not necessarily whole.)
- [ ] Pumpernickel
- [ ] Rice
- [ ] Rice flour
- [ ] Rye flour or rye
- [ ] Stone-ground wheat (If whole grain, product should say "stone ground *whole* wheat.")
- [ ] Wheat
- [ ] Wheat flour
- [ ] Wheat germ (While not a whole grain, wheat germ is still good for you.)
- [ ] Unbleached wheat flour

- Look for *whole* on the ingredient list. If you see *whole-wheat*, or *whole-rye*, then it's clear the food contains whole grain. See opposite page.
- Look at where the whole grain falls in the ingredient list. Remember, foods are listed in order of weight, starting with the heaviest. If a whole grain is the only grain listed, then yes, you've got lots of whole grain in that bread, cracker, or pasta. But often you'll see *wheat flour* (white flour) as the first ingredient, followed by some sort of sweetener, then *whole-wheat flour*. In this case, whole grain is *not* the dominant grain; in fact, there might be just a trace amount.
- Look for components of whole wheat. For taste and texture reasons, some manufacturers split up the whole grain and reassemble it. Sounds convoluted, but you might have a product with all the nutrition of a whole grain with an ingredient list that reads "wheat flour, bran, wheat germ." You can't tell whether the product contains the same levels of bran and germ as the original amounts in the whole grain. However, these products are far healthier than foods made with white flour, so go for them.
- Check dietary fiber. In general, 100-percent whole-grain bread should have at least 2 g fiber per ounce (29 g) or per 80 calories; crackers at least 3 g fiber per ounce; pasta at least 5 g fiber per 2 ounces dried.
- Beware of the label claim *Made with whole grain*. That might mean that a little whole grain is thrown in but white flour is usually the primary ingredient.

7

Slender Shopping: An Aisle-by-Aisle Supermarket Tour

Ever found yourself stuck at the cereal aisle, mesmerized and overwhelmed by the choices? Wouldn't it be great to have a nutritionist at your side, pointing out just what to buy? That's what you get in this chapter, a guided tour of the supermarket aisles where you'll put your new label-reading skills to work. You'll see real brand name examples of what to—and not to—buy. But even better, you get guidelines to help you figure out for yourself the best foods of any brand. Next time you walk into a supermarket, you'll shun the sodium and saturated-fat–drenched foods, and fill your cart with slimming, healthful (and delicious) groceries. (Manufacturers change formulations periodically, so you may find differences from some of the nutritional information here.)

In appendix 2 on page 261, you can photocopy or tear out pages that summarize the recommended nutritional guidelines for cereal, frozen dinners, and other staples. (You'll also find the same information on the *Good Housekeeping* website at www.goodhousekeeping.com, which you can download and print.)

Before you head down the aisles, a few overall tips and strategies:

- *Bring a list.* In the sanity of your own home, away from the cheese curls and fudge sticks, make a list of items you need that's based on *The Supermarket Diet* meals. Stick to your list as closely as possible.
- *Bring a calculator.* You'll need it to compare the nutritional value of brands with different serving sizes.
- *Buy the least-processed foods.* For instance, get plain rice instead of sodium-spiked flavored rice. The foods won't taste plain after you use the delicious recipes in this book! What they *will* lack: the excess sodium and unhealthy fats of processed foods.
- *Look for health foods.* Many mainstream supermarkets have a health food section. Ignore the health food cookies and chips (they might make you as fat as the regular stuff), but if you can afford it, buy the lower-sodium beans, the higher-fiber/lower-sugar cereal, the vegetarian chili, the whole-grain frozen waffles, and other healthful foods.
- *Avoid the chip, soda, and cookie aisles.* Remember: If you can get into your car without them, then they won't be tempting you at home. If you have a craving later on, then make a special trip to a bakery or a convenience store and buy just one cookie, one small bag of chips, one soda, or one serving of whatever it is you're craving.
- *Don't focus solely on calories.* Sure, chicken noodle soup isn't a high-calorie food. But it's usually loaded with sodium, and for many people, too much sodium raises blood pressure. Sodium, saturated fat, and trans fat are all linked to heart disease and other ills. You want to minimize these substances, especially if you're overweight, which itself is a risk factor for disease. Thanks to your label reading, you'll figure out which chicken noodle soup is lowest in sodium. By comparing labels you'll pick brands with less of the bad stuff and more of the good stuff, like fiber, vitamins, and minerals.
- *Remind yourself of the recommended levels of nutrients for your plan* (see "Recommended Daily Intakes" on page 160). Jot the information down and stick it in your wallet (or download it from the *Good Housekeeping* website at www.goodhousekeeping.com). Then, when you're in the market and staring at a cereal label, wondering whether 13 g is a little or a lot of sugar for a serving (it's a lot!), you can pull out your cheat sheet and see that 24 g added sugars is your maximum allowed for the entire day on the 1,500-calorie Keep On Losin' plan.

- *Remember, ingredients are listed by weight.* The first ingredient is the heaviest (usually the most by volume as well), followed by the next heaviest, and so on. So, if the first ingredient in a cereal or bread is "enriched flour" or "wheat flour," watch out; it might be mainly white flour! (See page 164 for a refresher on how to spot whole grains in any ingredient list.)
- *Get the freshest foods.* Ask the produce guys, the fishmonger, even the meat and poultry people on which days foods come in. If it jives with your schedule, shop on those days.
- *Go alone.* If possible, don't take the kids or anyone else who'll try to get you to buy foods you don't need.
- *Don't shop when you're hungry.* You've heard this before but just remember: Shopping when you're full truly cuts down on fattening impulse buys!

As you shop, you may wonder if health foods are better. Here's the deal: There are more healthful foods to choose from in a big health food or natural foods supermarket than in a mainstream grocery store (unless that grocery store has a well-stocked health food section.) Health food stores tend to stock more foods rich in whole grain, fiber, and vegetables than do mainstream markets. And, for the most part, there's less sugar, sodium, trans fat, and nitrates (a preservative). For instance, you've got more high-fiber/low-sugar cereals to choose from in a health food store. The canned beans and other canned goods tend to be lower in sodium. The crackers and cookies are not made with trans fat (although mainstream companies are starting to get the trans fat out of their products as well).

The catch? Price. You pay for the healthier stuff. Sometimes a lot more, sometimes just pennies more. The Whole Foods (a large natural foods supermarket) house brand—365—is priced competitively with mainstream brands. But you may not have a Whole Foods near you, or even a small health food store. In that case, there should be enough mainstream brands that fit the guidelines in this chapter; you just won't have as many choices. Another option: Order some of those foods from the grocery websites.

Beware: There's also a lot of health food junk food! Chips, even if fried in canola oil, are still a high-cal/low-nutrient food. And trans fat–free cookies are still full of sugar and calories and low in vitamins.

Fruit-juice-sweetened sodas are still loaded with empty calories. (By the time a fruit juice is boiled down to become a sweetener, it's lost most of its nutrition.) So, while health food stores or health food sections of supermarkets carry a lot of great products, don't be fooled by the seemingly healthier foods that can undermine your weight loss.

Ready, set, SHOP!

Start Here: The Produce Section

Go ahead and splurge! Everything's fair game! It's all healthful and slimming. Your main goals: taste, price, and getting a wide enough variety.

The tastiest and least expensive produce is usually what's in season. Peaches and tomatoes are lusciously tasty in late summer but bland or mealy in winter. Or you pay crazy-expensive prices for out-of-season imports from South America and elsewhere, where the produce is in season.

While the produce area can sometimes be overwhelming with weird-looking fruits and vegetables you've never even heard of, fight the temptation to pick up the same old bananas and romaine lettuce. Being more adventurous not only makes for more interesting meals but also helps keep you healthier. That's because different fruits and vegetables have different types of health-promoting nutrients; the more variety in your diet the more nutrients you score. *The Supermarket Diet* meals offer a wide variety. You can widen it even more by substituting fruits or vegetables of your choice in our meal plans.

One way to ensure that you take in the full spectrum of vitamins, minerals, and other beneficial compounds (called *phytonutrients*) is by eating produce of different colors. Here's what you get when you take the rainbow approach:

Green

Outstanding nutrients: Lutein and zeaxanthin, powerful antioxidants (especially lutein) linked to a reduced risk of two eye diseases: cataracts and macular degeneration, the leading cause of blindness.

Found in: Asparagus, beet greens, broccoli, Brussels sprouts, collard greens, dandelion greens, green beans, honeydew melon, kale, kiwi, mustard greens, okra, parsley, peas, peppers, spinach, Swiss chard, romaine lettuce, zucchini.

Outstanding nutrient: Vitamin K, critical for proper wound healing and for strong bones.
  Found in: Beet greens, broccoli, Brussels sprouts, collard greens, dandelion greens, endive, kale, mustard greens, parsley, spinach, Swiss chard, turnip greens.

Outstanding nutrients: Cancer-fighting compounds called *indoles* and *isothiocyanates* are abundant in cruciferous vegetables.
  Found in: Arugula, bok choy, broccoflower (a broccoli and cauliflower hybrid), broccoli, Brussels sprouts, cabbage (all types), cauliflower, collard greens, kale, mustard greens, rutabaga, Swiss chard, turnip greens, turnips, watercress.

Yellow/Orange

Outstanding nutrients: Beta and alpha carotene, antioxidants that are linked to a reduced risk of cancer and heart disease, are the hallmark of orange-hued fruits and veggies.
  Found in: Apricots, butternut squash, cantaloupe, carrots, mangoes, peaches, pumpkin, sweet potatoes.

The Butter Fruit: Avocados

Everything green in the produce section is good for you. But just one note about avocados: Think of them as a fat instead of a vegetable. While they are a healthy fat—rich in heart-healthy monounsaturated fat—they are also high calorie, like all fats. An eighth of a Hass avocado has about the same calorie and fat content as a teaspoon of margarine, butter, or oil. You don't need to avoid avocados; just stick to one-fourth of a fruit or less to keep calories in check. Avocados are a rich source of B vitamins, good for the heart and brain.

Outstanding nutrients: Bioflavonoids and vitamin C. Oranges and grapefruit contain citrus bioflavonoids, which may help protect against cancer and heart disease. Citrus peel contains limonene, which helps fight cancer.

Found in: Apricots, clementines, grapefruit, lemons, limes, nectarines, oranges, papaya, peaches, pears, pineapple, tangerines, yellow peppers.

Outstanding nutrient: Potassium, which helps protect against heart disease.

Found in: Apricots, bananas, grapefruit, lemons, oranges, pineapple.

Red

Outstanding nutrient: Lycopene is a powerful antioxidant linked to protection from cancer and heart disease and gives foods their red color.

Found in: Pink grapefruit, red tomatoes, salsa, tomato-based juices, tomato-based pasta sauce, tomato soup, watermelon.

Purple/Blue/Deep Red

Outstanding nutrients: Anthocyanins, a potent group of antioxidants, help prevent blood clots and may improve brain function.

Found in: Blueberries, cherries, cranberries, eggplant, grape juice, plums, prunes (dried plums), raisins, red apples, red beans, red beets, red cabbage, red or purple grapes, red onions, red pears, red wine, strawberries.

White/Pale Green

Outstanding nutrients: Allyl sulfides, which help prevent stomach and colon cancer and may lower cholesterol, are found in onions, potatoes, and especially garlic. Onions are also a good source of quercitin, which protects against cancer and, possibly, heart disease. The rest contain flavonoids, a large class of phytochemicals linked to protection against heart disease.

Found in: Artichokes, asparagus, celery, chives, endive, garlic, green pears, mushrooms, onions, scallions.

1 Aisle 1
Canned Poultry and Fish, Condiments, Salad Dressings, Sauces/Marinades

Canned Poultry and Fish

CHICKEN IN CAN OR POUCH
Perhaps this sounds a little odd, but canned chicken is surprisingly good in chicken salad, casseroles, or other mixed dishes. And chicken in cans or pouches has a plus over the refrigerated deli sliced chicken or turkey: no nitrites or nitrates, which, with regular use, may contribute to cancer. They're also a lot lower in sodium: For instance, 1 ounce of Valley Fresh White Chicken (canned) has 35 mg sodium and Tyson's Chicken Breast in a pouch has 105 mg, compared to about 300 mg sodium per ounce for some brands of refrigerated turkey breast deli slices.

SALMON IN CAN
Most brands use wild salmon, which, according to some research, has a lower likelihood of contamination with PCBs—a type of chemical that may contribute to cancer—than farm-raised salmon.

TUNA IN CAN OR POUCH
If tuna is a staple in your house, use more light tuna in water instead of white albacore to cut back on mercury. The tuna in pouches has a firmer consistency than the canned and now comes in a variety of flavors.

Condiments

HONEY
You'll need it on *The Supermarket Diet* to sweeten plain yogurt and smoothies, and you can also use honey on bread instead of jam or jelly. While honey does contain some phytonutrients (so it's better for you than sugar), just remember: It's 64 calories per tablespoon. So watch the portions.

JAM/JELLY

Go ahead and choose regular or lower-calorie jams or jellies; either one is fine. It all depends on how important jam and jelly is to you as a small calorie splurge. (If it's the only way you'll down a piece of high-fiber bread, it's pretty important!) Here's what's counted toward your 125-calorie treat allowance:

- Regular jam and jelly typically run about 50 to 55 calories per table-spoon, so if you like the real stuff, pick whatever brand or flavor you prefer.
- "Low-sugar" can cut calories in half without artificial sweeteners, as in Smucker's Low Sugar Strawberry Jam at 25 calories per tablespoon.
- "Sugar-free" does use artificial sweeteners. Thanks to aspartame (NutraSweet) Smucker's sugar-free strawberry is just 10 calories per tablespoon.

KETCHUP

All the brands are about 15 calories per tablespoon, with about 190 mg sodium and 4 g sugar. If you stick with a tablespoon, don't worry about calories. But if you're a real ketchup fiend, remember to subtract those extra ketchup calories from your treat allowance. Also, you might con-sider trying the reduced-sodium ketchups.

MUSTARDS

They're all low calorie, about 5 calories per teaspoon, so get the lowest-sodium brands you like. For instance, Gulden's Spicy Brown mustard is a good choice with 50 mg sodium per teaspoon; some other brands have as much as 100 mg or more.

PEANUT BUTTER AND OTHER NUT BUTTERS

The main difference among peanut butter brands is sodium. For instance, some brands have more than 200 mg sodium per tablespoon, others have closer to 150 mg and still others have no sodium at all. If you like a little salt, then buy the 120-mg brands. If you don't mind salt-free, even better.

Some commercial brands of peanut butter contain partially hydrogenated oil, but since their level of trans fat is under 0.5 g per serving (2 tablespoons), they can be reported as "0 g." That could mean there's as much as 0.49 g. If you want to be on the safe side and avoid trans completely, go with brands like Smucker's, Arrowhead Mills, or 365 (the Whole Foods label) that are simply nuts or nuts and salt, without added hydrogenated fat.

Skip the reduced-fat brands; they don't save any calories, because they pump the peanut butter up with fillers. Since the fat in peanut butter is a healthy fat, best to use the real stuff.

With a higher percentage of monounsaturated fat than peanut butter (which itself is no nutritional slouch and tends to be higher in protein than other nut butters), almond and cashew butter make a nice change.

You'll need to pick up tahini (ground sesame seeds) if you make the hummus on Friday, Week 2 of Boot Camp, or for one of the Keep On Losin' lunches. (Or, you can simply buy ready-made hummus if your store carries it.) In health food stores, tahini is stocked along with other nut butters; in supermarkets, you may have to look in the ethnic food aisles.

SOY SAUCE AND OTHER ASIAN SAUCES

Some recipes in this book call for reduced-sodium soy sauce and even then, for just a little bit. Here's why: Regular soy sauce has about 1,260 mg sodium per tablespoon. That's more than half the 2,300 mg sodium daily cap! The light sauce is still sodium heavy, but you're not going to need the full tablespoon serving size on the label.

GUIDELINES FOR SOY SAUCE
▶ Serving size: 1 tablespoon
▶ Sodium: 560 mg or less

A great sauce for those limiting sodium is Sweet-and-Sour Sauce. Two tablespoons are 50 calories with just 60 mg sodium. It works as both a stir-fry sauce or a condiment for seasoning vegetables after they're cooked.

Salad Dressings

They're all over the nutritional map. The most important issues: taste, calories, and type of fat. Since calories vary from nearly nothing—15 calories for 2 tablespoons of some fat-free types—to 180 calories for 2

COMPARE THE LABELS: SALAD DRESSING			
	Newman's Own Olive Oil & Vinegar	Kraft Zesty Italian	Kraft Light Done Right! Zesty Italian
Ingredients	olive oil, vegetable oil (soybean oil and/or canola oil), water, red wine vinegar, onion, spices, salt, garlic, lemon juice, and distilled vinegar	canola and/or soybean oil, water, vinegar, salt, sugar, contains less than 2% of garlic*, garlic onion*, spice, lemon juice concentrate, etc.	water, vinegar, sugar, soybean and olive oil, salt, contains less than 2% of garlic*, garlic, xanthan gum, onions*, etc.
Serving size	2 tablespoons	2 tablespoons	2 tablespoons
Calories	150	80	25
Sodium	150 mg	310 mg	470 mg

Newman's Own scores best on sodium and has a higher percentage of "good" fat, because the first oil listed is olive oil. But both types of Kraft dressings are lower in calories. So, you have to decide what's more important to you: sodium or calories. Or you might luck out and find a dressing that's got both things going for it. At 150 calories (75 calories per tablespoon) the Newman's Own Dressing would fit into any of *The Supermarket Diet* menus that simply call for "salad dressing." But if you don't want to spend many of your calories on dressing, don't have high blood pressure, or will limit sodium in the rest of the meal, either Kraft dressing is fine. A possible compromise: See if you can get away with just 1 tablespoon of the Newman's Own or either of the Krafts. Or "stretch" the dressing with a little lemon juice or balsamic vinegar.

tablespoons Caesar, your choice depends on how you want to budget your calories. If the only way you'll eat salad is with a full-fat dressing, then that's the type for you. It's a good calorie investment. But if you like the low-calorie dressings just fine and would rather have another slice of bread with your meal, that's your prerogative.

GUIDELINES FOR SALAD DRESSINGS
- **Calories:** Regular dressing should be 100 to 150 calories per 2 tablespoons, the serving size usually listed on the label. That's what's allotted in *The Supermarket Diet* menus. You don't have to use 2 tablespoons. Start with one and go up from there if you must. Reduced-fat/reduced-calorie dressing will be under 100 calories per 2-tablespoon serving.
- **Fat:** Choose dressings with olive oil or canola oil. While soybean, corn, or peanut oil are OK once in a while, your mainstay salad dressing should have canola or olive oil, because of their healthy balance of monounsaturated and polyunsaturated oils.
- **Sodium:** Compare labels: Choose those lower in sodium.

Sauces/Marinades

Here you'll find sauces that transform plain meat, chicken, fish, or tofu into interesting main dishes. But watch it; generally, they're loaded with sodium.

GUIDELINE FOR SAUCES
Always go for the product lowest in sodium. Label sleuthing can save you hundreds of milligrams of sodium. Be sure to compare products of equivalent amounts.

COMPARE THE LABELS: BOTTLED SAUCES		
	Brand A **worcestershire sauce**	**Brand B steak sauce**
Serving size	1 teaspoon	1 tablespoon
Calories	5	15
Sodium	65 mg	280 mg

Did you catch the difference in serving size? To compare fairly, let's figure out what's in a tablespoon of Brand A worcestershire sauce by multiplying a teaspoon by three, since there are 3 teaspoons in 1 tablespoon. There are 15 calories—the same as Brand B steak sauce—and 195 mg sodium, nearly 100 mg *less* than Brand B. Clearly, Brand A is the better bet here.

Aisle 2

Canned Beans, Canned Broth, Canned Soup, Canned Vegetables, Chili, Pasta, Pasta Sauce, Rice and Other Grains

Canned Beans

They're a staple in all *The Supermarket Diet* plans because beans are high in fiber, which leaves you feeling full for a good while—and chock full of vitamins and minerals. All types are good for you. The only issue here is sodium, which typically runs from 250 to 500 mg per ½ cup. Rinsing beans with tap water removes lots of the sodium. Health food store brands tend to be much lower in sodium: about 140 mg per ½ cup. Eden Foods No Salt Added beans have an outstandingly low 25 to 35 mg sodium per ½ cup. A staple of health food markets, these beans are also appearing on conventional supermarket shelves.

Baked beans are fine, on occasion, but with 12 g sugar per ½ cup (compared to 0 g for plain beans), they cut way into your daily sugar allotment. If you can find them, Eden Foods Baked Beans cut sugar back to 6 g per ½ cup.

Your other option is to soak and cook dried beans, giving you control over the sodium. You'll usually find these in the rice aisle.

Canned Broth

The recipes in this book call for reduced-sodium broths. If your supermarket doesn't carry them, request that the store begin stocking them. The difference in sodium is staggering: For instance, Swanson's Lower Sodium Beef Broth has 390 mg sodium per cup versus 790 mg for the regular version. HerbOx Low Sodium Granulated Bouillon, either beef or chicken, has only 5 mg sodium per teaspoon or cube (each makes 1 cup broth).

GUIDELINE FOR BROTH
Look for brands with less than 400 mg sodium per cup.

Canned Soup

Think beans, and you're golden. Black bean, split pea, lentil, a bean-based minestrone can all be turned into super fiber-rich main courses. Skip the cream soups: too much fat and too few nutrients. Chicken noodle, chicken and rice, beef and vegetable (all the clear soups with a little meat, vegetables, and starch) aren't as nutritious as bean soups. However, if you love them, have 80 calories' worth (about 1 cup) and think of it as equivalent to a slice of bread or ½ cup rice or pasta. In other words, forgo one of your starch servings in the meal if you're going to have a cup of chicken noodle or similar soup.

Canned Vegetables

Fresh or frozen usually taste better than canned and are more nutritious. However, canned, no-sodium added, vacuum-packed corn or canned tomatoes are great products that you'll find in *The Supermarket Diet* recipes. Check the front of labels for "reduced sodium," or "no sodium added" to quickly spot the winners.

COMPARE THE LABELS: CANNED CORN		
	Brand A corn	Brand B no salt added corn
Serving size	$1/3$ cup	$1/3$ cup
Calories	80	60
Sodium	230 mg	0 mg
Sugar	5 g	2 g
Not only is the no salt product sodium-free, but it is also lower in calories because there is no sugar (a careful ingredient-reading discovery).		

Chili

Get bean-based chilis, either vegetarian chili or turkey/chicken chili. Beef chilis tend to be too high in saturated fat. Even the health food store chilis tend to be high in sodium, so watch your sodium intake carefully the rest of the day.

GUIDELINES FOR CANNED CHILI
- **Serving size:** 1 cup
- **Calories:** 210 or less
- **Saturated fat:** 1 g or less
- **Sodium:** 800 mg or less

Pasta

Look for whole-wheat pasta, which has a tremendous fiber advantage over regular pasta.

COMPARE THE LABELS: PASTA			
	Regular Pasta	Whole-Wheat Pasta (e.g., DeBoles, De Cecco Whole Wheat, organic whole-wheat pasta)	Ronzoni Healthy Harvest Whole Wheat Pasta Blend
Serving size	2 ounces	2 ounces	2 ounces
Calories	210	180 to 210	180
Dietary fiber	1 to 2 g	5 to 7 g	6 g

All three pastas are similar in calories, but whole-wheat pastas and Ronzoni have a lot more fiber because their main ingredient is whole wheat or, in the case of Ronzoni Healthy Harvest, wheat bran has been added to the white flour. Ronzoni doesn't offer quite as much vitamin E as a whole-wheat pasta, but this is still an excellent choice, especially if you don't like the taste of whole-wheat pasta.

Pasta Sauce

Do yourself a favor and avoid fattening Alfredo and cheese sauces. Instead, explore the seemingly endless varieties of tomato sauces (or make your own, see page 118). You get twice as much red sauce as you would with the creamy Alfredo—½ cup—for just 70 to 80 calories. Plus you're getting the health-promoting properties of lycopene, a powerful antioxidant that gives tomatoes their red color.

GUIDELINES FOR RED SAUCE

Try to find a product that meets at least three out of the four nutritional values per 1/2 cup.

▶ **Serving size:** 1/2 cup
▶ **Calories:** 90 calories or less
▶ **Fat:** 4 g or less
▶ **Saturated fat:** 2 g or less
▶ **Sodium:** 600 mg or less

Keep your eye on sodium, which varies a lot, even within brands.

Rice and Other Grains

Start with plain rice and jazz it up yourself to save oodles of sodium over some of the prepackaged versions. If you add ¼ teaspoon salt (580 mg sodium) to 1 cup rice, once cooked, the rice expands to a little over 3 cups. That works out to about 194 mg sodium per cup compared to about 1,000 mg sodium for 1 cup Rice-A-Roni. Or cook it in a reduced-sodium broth and still come out way ahead on sodium. Add a little chopped parsley or cilantro and some toasted almonds or pine nuts, and you've got a tasty creation. However, if you like the convenience of rice mixes, scrutinize labels for the lower-sodium varieties. The Near East brand, found in both mainstream and health food groceries, has tasty rice, couscous, and mixed-grain boxed mixes for under 600 mg sodium per serving. Not low but better than 1,000 mg! Rice-A-Roni does carry a "⅓ less salt" product, which is a better bet than the regular.

Even if you love white rice, give brown rice a try. It's got more fiber than white and more phytonutrients (beneficial plant compounds). If you don't have the 40 minutes it takes to make brown, there's Uncle Ben's Ready Rice, which microwaves in 90 seconds. Get adventurous, there are some unusual, beautiful, and very tasty whole-grain rices. If you can get your hands on it, buy Texmati brown rice or Lundberg Family Farms brown jasmine rice or any brand of brown basmati rice, all fragrant, interesting varieties. Lundberg Family Farms (in health food markets and some mainstream groceries) also makes Organic Black Japonica, a blend of black rice (!) and mahogany rice. Cooking rice in a low-sodium chicken broth adds flavor. Near East offers flavored mixes that combine brown rice with barley and wheat, with substantial amounts of fiber. Compare labels and choose those lowest in sodium.

Try to break your routine and eat grains other than rice, such as bulgur wheat and whole-wheat couscous, quinoa (a little, round, whole grain from South America), barley (loaded with cholesterol-lowering soluble fiber), buckwheat, and amaranth (actually a vegetable, not a grain, that's made into pasta and cereal). You can probably find most of these—certainly barley—in the supermarket.

3 Aisle 3
Breakfast Bars, Cereal, Cocoa, and Coffee and Tea

Breakfast Bars

Most so-called breakfast bars aren't worth it: too much sugar and too little fiber. But keep looking; there is the occasional decent offering, such as All Bran bars (130 calories, 5 g fiber). Or jump over to the energy-bar shelf and pick up an Odwalla Bar with at least 4 g fiber, such as Superfood or Cranberry C Monster. Keep bars around in case there's no time for breakfast, or as an emergency meal at the office (but don't make it a habit; they're not nutritionally balanced enough to constitute "breakfast").

Cereal

COLD CEREAL

It's a dizzying array, but armed with these guidelines, you'll pick a good cold cereal. Kashi GoLean (not GoLean Crunch) is a great choice. With 10g fiber per 140 calories, it exceeds the guidelines, and it is also low in sugar and saturated fat.

HIGHER-PROTEIN CEREALS

The fronts of many cereal boxes not only boast of fiber content but also now advertise grams of protein, usually derived from soy. Some of my clients find the higher-protein cereals more satisfying, keeping them feeling full all the way to lunch in contrast to the lack of staying power of lower-protein cereals. Try out a higher-protein cereal for yourself. Look for 8 g protein per 100 calories or 16 per 150 calories. Kashi GoLean fits the bill. So does Kellogg's Special K for a Low-Carb Lifestyle, with a whopping 10g protein per 100 calories, lots of fiber (8g) and very little sugar. Another plus: Soy protein has been proven to help lower cholesterol (in conjunction with a diet low in saturated and trans fat).

HOT CEREALS

Hot cereals usually don't have as much fiber as the high-fiber cold cereals (because they're usually not boosted with added bran), but hot cereals are decent sources of fiber and, if you avoid the sugary ones, a very nutritious breakfast staple. In general, when it comes to choosing a hot cereal, the chewier the better. That's because the coarser the grain the longer it takes to digest and turn into blood sugar. A slow transformation to blood sugar can help suppress appetite. For example, steel-cut oats that take 15 minutes to digest are probably more helpful to your weight loss than instant oats. The 5-minute oats are somewhere in between. All oats are whole grain; some are more or less processed. But if all you have time for is instant, then no problem; they're still healthful.

GUIDELINES FOR HOT CEREALS

▶ **Ingredient list:** 100% whole grain or whole grain plus bran and/or wheat germ. Examples of whole grains in the ingredient list: barley, brown rice, oats, quinoa, whole rye, whole triticale, whole wheat. Exception: Oat bran: It's just the bran, not the whole-grain oat, but it's been proven to help lower cholesterol, so if you like it, go for it.

▶ **Sugar:** Less than 5 g per 100 calories

▶ **Fiber:** At least 4 g per 150 calories

COMPARE THE LABELS: OATMEAL

	Brand A (instant)	Brand B (lower sugar)	Brand C (plain)
Ingredients	whole-grain rolled oats (with oat bran), sugar, natural and artificial flavors, salt, calcium carbonate, guar gum, caramel color, etc.	whole-grain rolled oats (with oat bran), sugar, natural and artificial flavors, salt, calcium carbonate, guar gum, caramel color, sucralose (Splenda® brand), etc.	100% natural rolled oats
Serving size	1 packet (43 g)	1 packet (34 g)	$1/2$ cup dry (40 g)
Calories	160	120	150
Sodium	270 mg	270 mg	0 mg
Total carbohydrates	33 g	24 g	27 g
Dietary fiber	3 g	3 g	4 g
Sugars	13 g	4 g	1 g

Ideally, you should buy the last one, the plain oatmeal. You get more oats, more fiber, and no sodium for fewer calories than from either of the other choices. Adding a teaspoon of maple syrup to the plain oats adds just 17 calories and 4 g sugar. You probably won't need much more than a teaspoon, especially if you throw in some fruit. However, if you really love the preflavored mixes, then the lower-sugar variety is probably best.

COMPARE THE LABELS: WHICH HOT CEREALS ARE MADE FROM WHOLE GRAIN?

	Brand A	Brand B	Brand C	Brand D
Ingredients	Wheat farina, wheat germ, disodium phosphate (for quick cooking), vitamins and minerals	100% natural rolled whole wheat	hard red wheat	toasted crushed wheat, wheat bran, wheat germ, and calcium carbonate
Serving size	33 g	1/2 cup dry (40 g)	1/4 cup (43 g)	1/3 cup (41 g)
Calories	120	130	150	160
Sodium	90 mg	0 mg	0 mg	0 mg
Total carbohydrates	25 g	30 g	32 g	33 g
Dietary fiber	1 g	4 g	2 g	5 g
Sugars	0 g	0 g	0 g	0 g

Brand B is a whole-wheat product, clearly stated on the label. Brands A and C don't specify "whole wheat" and with their low fiber numbers, they are not whole-grain products. The Brand D label is more confusing: Is "toasted crushed wheat" whole wheat or not? A call to the manufacturer revealed that yes, it is whole wheat, plus the extra bran and germ. (See "How to Spot the Whole Grain in the Ingredients List," page 164.) And the fiber content is right up there with Brand B.

Cocoa

A cup of hot cocoa or cold chocolate milk made with fat-free milk is an excellent choice for your daily snack or your daily calcium treat. Good news: Cocoa powder is rich in heart-healthy compounds. Depending on your tastes and where you prefer to budget calories, here are your choices:

- *Unsweetened cocoa powder.* Two teaspoons (8 calories) plus another 2 teaspoons sugar (33 calories), a dash of vanilla extract (3 calories), and 1 cup fat-free milk (86 calories) come to 130 calories.
- *Sweetened cocoa powder.* Brands vary. For instance, 1½ tablespoons Ghirardelli Sweet Ground Chocolate and Cocoa (45 calories) with a cup of fat-free milk is 131 calories. (The Ghirardelli label lists the serving size as 3 tablespoons, but you don't need that much.) Nesquick Chocolate mix is another good choice at 45 calories per tablespoon.
- *Add-water complete cocoa mixes.* They range from just 25 or 50 calories for the no-sugar varieties (e.g., Swiss Miss No Sugar Added) to about 170 calories for those with sugar (as in Hershey's Hot Cocoa Mix "Dutch Chocolate" flavor.) If you use these, stick with no more than 150 calories per envelope and make sure they're calcium-enriched with at least 25 percent DV for calcium per envelope. Otherwise you're missing out on the biggest nutritional benefit to hot chocolate: the calcium!

Coffee and Tea

Although there are no caffeine restrictions on *The Supermarket Diet,* it's probably a good idea to limit coffee to no more than 2 cups daily and tea to 4 or 5 cups. Tea drinkers have lower rates of heart disease, and while studies show that 1 or 2 cups of coffee per day is fine, some studies suggest that heavy coffee drinking (5 cups per day) can raise blood sugar, particularly in people with hypertension (high blood pressure). Buy plain tea or coffee instead of sugary chai or coffee drinks, or flavored coffee powders that are high in sugar and fat. You have more control when you add your own sugar: just 16 calories per teaspoon. For instance, steeping Tazo Chai tea in a cup of hot water and adding 1 teaspoon sugar and 2 tablespoons 2% milk totals 31 calories. Made with a concentrated chai mix, you're looking at about 80 to 200 calories per cup. An envelope of some powdered instant capuccinos could hit you with 90 calories and 18 g sugar. And a 9.5-

ounce bottle of a cold cappuccino could have as many as 170 calories and a whopping 30 g sugar. Make a skim-milk cappuccino with a shot of espresso or a teaspoon of instant espresso powder (1 calorie), 6 ounces skim milk (64 calories, 4 g sugar) and a shot of sugar-free vanilla syrup (0 calories), and you've saved lots of calories and sugar grams, and gained some calcium.

Aisle 4
Bagels and English Muffins, Bread, and Crackers

Bagels and English Muffins

If a bagel or English muffin is whole grain—whole wheat or multigrain without white flour—then you may substitute it for whole-grain bread. However, there are very few nationally available whole-grain English muffins or bagels. And even if you find a 100 percent whole-grain bagel, there's a catch: Bagels are generally huge, with three to five times more calories than a slice of bread. So, half a bagel is equivalant to two slices of bread which can be a little frustrating for some people.

A few nationally distributed companies also make 100% whole-wheat English muffins, but they might be hard to find in the grocery store. Don't be fooled by English muffins that sound whole grain–rich, but might not be. They might even use words like "multi-grain" and "wheat" in their names. (See box on page 164 to find out what ingredients to look for on the nutrition label to make sure you are getting whole wheat.) In some cases where the first ingredient is white flour, they may have only 2 g fiber for 140 calories. For that number of calories you'd get 3–4 g fiber from 100 percent whole-wheat bread. If you find a 100 percent whole-wheat English muffin, go for it, and remember: It's the equivalent of two slices of bread. You might try Pepperidge Farm English Muffins 100% Whole Wheat with 3 g fiber for 130 calories, or Orowheat 100% Whole Wheat English Muffins (available west of the Mississippi) with 4 g fiber for 130 calories.

Bread

As explained throughout this book, a high-fiber diet will help you lose weight and protect you from a host of chronic diseases. Since whole-grain bread is a good source of fiber, it's recommended throughout *The Supermarket Diet* menus. White bread is OK as an occasional treat, though your mainstay should be whole grain/high fiber. But with all the choices—multigrain, cracked wheat, wheat, oatmeal, and pumpernickel—how do you begin to figure out what to buy? Since the name of a product can be misleading ("Honey Wheat English Muffins" sound wholesome, but they've actually got very little whole wheat), go straight to the ingredient list and the nutrition facts panel.

> **GUIDELINES FOR BREAD**
> ▶ Choose 100 percent whole wheat (or other whole grain)
> ▶ **Calories:** 60 to 75 per slice
> ▶ **Dietary fiber:** at least 2 g per ounce (29 g). For many breads, 1 ounce is about 1 slice.
> ▶ **Ingredient list:** The first ingredient should be a whole grain, with the word *whole* in front of the words *wheat, rye,* or another grain. Oats don't have to be preceded by *whole.* Also acceptable: a white-flour product with bran and germ added back, such as Arnold's Branola (this one is 90 calories per slice, too high for Boot Camp and Keep On Losin', but OK for the Stay Slim Maintenance plan).
>
> A note about "light" bread. These breads have 40 to 45 calories per slice, about half as much as regular bread. Choose those made primarily with whole wheat, offering 2 g fiber per slice (as in Arnold Bakery Light Whole Wheat). If you substitute light bread for regular in this book, you're left with about 60 extra calories to play with.

Crackers

Crackers are rife with misleading labels. The word *wheat* in the name and wholesome-looking packaging makes a lot of crackers appear to be made with whole grain, but most aren't. Again, like bread, look at the ingredient list and find the fiber in the nutrition facts panel.

GUIDELINES FOR CRACKERS, per ounce
▶ **Serving size:** 1 ounce (29 g)
▶ **Calories:** 115 to 130
▶ **Dietary fiber:** at least 3 g
▶ **Saturated fat:** 0.5 or less
▶ **Sodium:** 200 mg or less (Ideally, but this may be hard to find, so if you've got the other elements in place, it's OK to exceed 200 mg.)
▶ **Ingredient list:** As with bread, the first ingredient should be a whole grain, with the word *whole* in front of the words *wheat, rye,* or another grain. Oats don't have to be preceded by *whole*. Also acceptable: a white-flour product with bran and germ added back.

Here are some good crackers, presented as a 1-ounce serving, along with their first four ingredients and the relevant nutrition info:

Ak Mak "Whole of the Wheat" Sesame Cracker
Ingredients: 100% stone ground "Whole of the Wheat" flour, water, clover honey, sesame oil, dairy butter
Serving size: 5 crackers, 1 ounce (28 g)
Calories: 116
Sodium: 200 mg
Total carbohydrates: 19 g
Dietary fiber: 3.5 g

Triscuit
Ingredients: Whole wheat, soybean oil, salt, monoglycerides
Serving size: 1 ounce (28 g)
Calories: 120
Sodium: 180 g
Total carbohydrates: 19 g
Dietary fiber: 3 g

Aisle 5

Frozen Burgers, Frozen Meals, Frozen Pizza, Frozen Soups, Frozen Vegetables, and Frozen Waffles

Frozen Burgers

FISH BURGERS AND FILLETS

There's trial and error involved in finding fresh-tasting, un-fishy frozen fish. The main reason for the fishy taste: At some point between leaving the factory and getting to your kitchen, the temperature dropped, causing the product to thaw slightly. While this isn't dangerous if you cook it thoroughly, the food loses some appeal. To maximize your chances of a fresh-tasting product:

- Gently squeeze the box. If it sounds and feels crunchy, put it back. That crunch is ice crystals, a sign of thaw and re-freeze.
- Pick boxes at the back of the freezer, especially if you're drawing from an open freezer. The back is colder.
- Adhere to the sell-by date.

Any fish is a nutritious choice as long as it's not breaded, fried, or encased in a fatty sauce. Buzzwords to look for: *grilled* or *unbreaded* or just plain, raw patties. As with poultry, some burgers or fillets are cooked then frozen, others frozen raw. Follow cooking instructions carefully to be safe.

Salmon is a fattier, therefore more caloric, fish than flounder, pollack, or other white fish. But some manufacturers remove much of the fat, where the stronger fishy flavors are embedded. So, many of the frozen salmon products are lower in calories and fat than fresh cuts. Still, the fat that's left is a good source of omega-3s, which are linked to lower risk of heart disease, depression, and alleviation of arthritis symptoms.

GUIDELINES FOR UNBREADED FISH FILLETS

These guidelines are a little loose, because numbers vary depending on the type of fish.

- **Serving size:** 3.8 ounces (108 g)
- **Calories:** Around 110
- **Fat:** Around 3 g
- **Saturated fat:** Around 0.5 g
- **Protein:** Around 17 g

GUIDELINES FOR FISH BURGERS

These guidelines are averages because precise numbers vary depending on the type of fish.

- **Serving size:** 3.2 ounces (91 g)
- **Calories:** Around 100
- **Fat:** Around 3 g
- **Saturated fat:** 0 to 1 g
- **Protein:** Around 17 g

CHICKEN AND TURKEY BURGERS

Frozen burgers (patties) or fillets come in very handy when you can't make it to the supermarket to get the fresh versions. Some are raw, some cooked; read the cooking instructions carefully. Most breaded patties or fillets are loaded with calories. There may be a few exceptions, however; read the labels carefully. (Avoid beef burgers because most are too high in calories and saturated fat.)

GUIDELINES FOR CHICKEN AND TURKEY BURGERS

- **Serving size:** 4 ounces (113 g)
- **Calories:** 160 to 170
- **Fat:** 8 g or less
- **Saturated fat:** 2.5 g or less
- **Protein:** 21 g or more

Compare those numbers to a breaded product, such as one that has the following per patty: 240 calories, 17 g fat, 3.5 g saturated fat, and just 8 g protein for a smaller, 76-g burger.

FROZEN VEGETABLE BURGERS

These come in two basic types: soy-based or vegetable/grain–based. While both are healthful products, *The Supermarket Diet* meals call for the soy-based, which are higher in protein and work beautifully as a substitute for chicken, meat, or other animal protein.

GUIDELINES FOR VEGETABLE BURGERS

▶ **Serving size:** 1 patty, about 2.5 ounces (70 g)
▶ **Calories:** Preferably 110 to 120 (If you like one of the lower-calorie burgers, such as Boca Original Burger for 70 calories, then have 1¹/₂ burgers.)
▶ **Protein:** 12 g or more
▶ **Sodium:** Preferably under 400 mg, but if all the other elements are in place, it's OK to exceed this.
▶ **Ingredient list:** Soy should be the first or second ingredient.

Frozen Meals

Despite the staggering number of frozen meals out there, there's a problem: The nutritionally balanced ones are often too low in calories. For instance, it's impressive that some brands of frozen foods include whole-wheat pasta and other whole-grain products, but you'll hear your stomach growling an hour after eating one of the 240- to 280-calorie meals. And then many of the calorically adequate meals have lackluster nutrition stats. For instance, one brand of frozen roasted chicken and stuffing may have the right number of calories (460) for a Keep On Losin' dinner (accompanied by some fruit for dessert or a little salad), but may also have more than 1000 mg sodium, very little fiber, a high amount of saturated fat, and no vegetables. Keep in mind that a balanced meal runs along these lines: at least 1 cup vegetables; ½ to 1 cup pasta, rice, or other grain; and about ¾ cup beans or 3 ounces animal protein.

You have three choices: find frozen meals with enough calories; get the low-calorie packages (Lean Cuisine's Spa Cuisine is a good choice) and bolster them with other foods, such as salad, a glass of milk, a little grated cheese, frozen vegetables, tofu, leftover chicken, and/or fruit for dessert; or, if a meal is only 240 or 250 calories, then have two for dinner (if you're on the Keep On Losin' plan) or two for lunch or dinner (if you're on the Maintenance plan.)

GUIDELINES FOR FROZEN MEALS

▶ **Calories:** 300 to 400 calories. Follow the suggestions above to bring meals up to a satisfying calorie level.

Look for products that meet at least two of the following criteria:
▶ **Saturated fat:** No more than 5 g
▶ **Fiber:** 5 g or more
▶ **Sodium:** 600 mg or less
▶ **Protein:** At least 14 g
▶ **Carbs:** Not much more than 45 g

COMPARE THE LABELS: FROZEN LASAGNA

	Brand A cheese lasagna	Brand B vegetable lasagna	Brand C tofu lasagna
Serving size	11.5 ounces (entire meal)	10.25 ounces (entire meal)	9.5 ounces (entire meal)
Calories	330	290	300
Saturated fat	3 g	4 g	1.5 g
Total carbohydrates	48 g	41 g	41 g
Dietary fiber	4 g	5 g	6 g
Protein	18 g	13 g	13 g
Sodium	690 mg	720 mg	630 mg
Vitamin A	10% DV	70% DV	60% DV
Vitamin C	10% DV	60% DV	35% DV
Calcium	30% DV	25% DV	10% DV
Iron	10% DV	15% DV	25% DV

These lasagna products don't differ all that much, and not one of them meets all the guidelines. But which one comes closest? It's a tie between Brand A and Brand C. Brand C meets the calorie, total carbohydrate, fiber, and saturated-fat guidelines. Brand A lasagna meets the calorie, sat-fat, and protein guidelines, and comes close enough to the total carbohydrate cutoff. Now, look more carefully at these two products: You'll see that Brand C has a superior vitamin content. But either one would be a good choice. To bring calories up, add a salad with regular dressing, and a fruit for dessert.

Frozen Pizza

Do pizza right—topped with vegetables, maybe some chicken—and you've got a tasty main course, moderate in calories, offering a serving of vegetables and substantial amounts of the powerful antioxidant lycopene, found in the tomato-based pizza sauce. But do it wrong—a pizza loaded with double cheese, pepperoni, sausage, and other meats—and you've got a calorie fiasco dripping with heart-unhealthy saturated fat.

GUIDELINES FOR PIZZA

▶ **Calories:** 450 to 470. That's a dinner portion on the Keep On Losin' plan. Add a salad with $1/2$ teaspoon olive oil—another 45 calories— for a meal total of about 500 calories. (If you want pizza for lunch on the Keep On Losin' plan, have about 350 calories' worth.) Read labels very carefully, sometimes 450 calories is an entire small pizza, sometimes a third of a pizza, or another amount. Do the math!

▶ **Saturated fat:** 7 g or less per 450 calories, which works out to be about 2 g saturated fat per 100 calories.

▶ **Sodium:** Compare labels. The lower the better!

▶ **Toppings:** vegetables, chicken, ham. Don't even pick up pizzas with pepperoni, sausage, ground beef, or double cheese. An exception: reduced-calorie pizzas, such as some of the Lean Cuisine Café Classics Pizzas, which manage to include pepperoni and sausage and keep saturated fat and calories low.

Here are two examples of within-guideline pizzas, and an example of one pizza that will require some side dishes to get up to the meal's full calorie requirement.

	Brand A Thai chicken	Brand B grilled chicken	Brand C spinach and mushroom
Serving size	1/3 pizza (123 g)	1/5 pizza (133 g)	1 pizza (175 g)
Calories	290	260	310
Fat	10 g	8 g	7 g
Saturated fat	3 g	3.5 g	3.5 g
Sodium	740 mg	550 mg	430 mg
Calcium	10% DV	20% DV	10% DV
Vitamin A	24% DV	10% DV	20% DV

You can have more than a third of the Brand A pizza. Actually, half the pizza comes to about 450 calories, 40 percent of the pizza works out to your 350 calories. Notice the ample amount of vitamin A, a nutrient bonus to vegetable-topped pizzas.

You can have more than the one-fifth serving size of the Brand B pizza; you get a third of the pizza for 450 calories. For 350 calories, you can have a little more than a quarter of the pizza. This one's lower in vitamin A than the first one but higher in calcium.

Brand C's pizza is so low in calories that you'll either have to break into a second one or include extra food in your meal. For a Keep On Losin' lunch of 400 calories, throw 3 tablespoons garbanzo or other beans in your salad and get another 50 calories. To bring calories up to the Keep On Losin' dinner level of 500 calories, have 1½ pizzas.

Frozen Soups

Look for Tabatchnick, a national brand. Most of its frozen soups are under 450 mg sodium, and many are high in fiber and nutrients.

Frozen Vegetables

As with fresh produce, think "variety." Either get a bag of mixed vegetables, or separate bags of broccoli, green and red peppers, etc., just as long as you're not buying all one type. Remember, cruciferous vegetables—broccoli, Brussels sprouts, cabbage, cauliflower, kale—are loaded with cancer-fighting compounds, so look for mixes that include these vegetables. Edamame (young green soybeans) and frozen spinach are other good choices. The plain vegetables have virtually no sodium and are easily doctored up by sautéing them in a little olive oil and garlic (thaw a little first), throwing them in a pasta sauce, or layering in a casserole. If you're not planning to cook, then go ahead and buy vegetables with sauce packets, comparing labels for lower-sodium products (you can use two thirds of the packets and cut back on sodium). Avoid most of the cheese sauce mixes: too much saturated fat and calories.

Frozen Waffles

Despite an astonishing number of frozen waffles, good luck finding one with even a speck of whole grain! The closest mainstream brand we found has a measly 3 g fiber for two waffles. No surprise when "enriched wheat flour" (white flour) tops the ingredients list, with "whole wheat" a distant third. However, health food stores really come through with a marvelous array of whole-grain waffles. For instance, several of Van's waffles (e.g., the Gourmet 97% Fat-Free or the Gourmet Multigrain) fit the guidelines below as do Kashi GoLean Waffles. The Kashi waffles have started appearing in mainstream supermarkets. Ask your grocer to stock them or another similar product.

Last Aisles: The Perimeters

Dairy, Deli Meats, Fresh Fish, Fresh Poultry, Fresh Meat, Hummus, Precooked Poultry, Smoked Salmon, and Tortillas

Make these your last stops on your shopping trip to help keep these perishables out of refrigeration for as short a time as possible.

Dairy

BUTTER/MARGARINE

The margarine versus butter debate seems to have finally ended, with trans fat–free margarine as the winner (see "Margarine or Butter?," page 89.) However, if you really love butter, use it; just stick with a few teaspoons a day, and use olive or canola oil to sauté foods. If you like your margarine unsalted, so much the better!

GUIDELINES FOR TRANS FAT–FREE MARGARINE

❱ **Serving size:** 1 tablespoon (14 g)
❱ **Calories:** 70 to 80
❱ **Total fat:** 8 to 9 g
❱ **Saturated fat:** 2.5 g or less
❱ **Trans fat:** 0 g
❱ **Sodium:** 95 g or less

CHEESE

The lower-priced, domestic cheeses are usually displayed separately from the fancier, imported, more expensive cheeses. You can stop at both stands. Reduced-fat domestic cheese (e.g., 2% Kraft Singles or

Cabot 50% Cheddar slices) is great for grilled cheese sandwiches or cheese toast for breakfast. Skip fat-free cheese; it tastes pretty terrible.

The fancier, more flavorful (and more caloric!) cheeses—blue cheese, gorgonzola, feta, Parmesan—serve more as condiments than as a main protein source in *Supermarket Diet* recipes. A little goes a long way. If you're a goat cheese fan, you're in luck; soft goat cheese is one of the lowest-calorie fancy cheeses. The softer the goat cheese, the fewer the calories. A hard goat cheese can run as high as 130 calories per ounce, a semisoft about 105, and the softest type a low 75 calories per ounce.

GUIDELINES FOR REDUCED-FAT/REDUCED-CALORIE CHEESE

▶ **Serving size:** 1 ounce (29 g)
▶ **Calories:** No more than 75
▶ **Fat:** No more than 4 g
▶ **Calcium:** At least 20% of the DV

CREAM CHEESE

Fortunately, reduced-fat cream cheese is a very satisfying spread, not too different in taste and feel from full fat. Full fat isn't worth the 200 calories per 2 tablespoons (the serving size usually listed on the label). And fat-free—even with a super-low 30 calories per 2 tablespoons—is just too grainy and weird.

GUIDELINES FOR REDUCED-FAT CREAM CHEESE

▶ **Serving size:** 2 tablespoons (30 g)
▶ **Calories:** 60 to 70
▶ **Fat:** 4 to 5 g
▶ **Saturated fat:** 3 g

EGGS

Supermarket Diet recipes or meals involving eggs use large eggs. If you can afford them, splurge on omega-3–enriched eggs. You'll see *omega 3* or *DHA* (a type of omega-3) on the label. These eggs not only provide 100 mg of this healthy fat, but some also are a little lower in cholesterol.

HUMMUS

This Middle Eastern spread is popping up in cold shelving in mainstream grocery stores, so you might not have to go to a health food store or ethnic market to find it. (Or, make your own. It's not hard, as you'll see on page 68.) Since there's not one standard recipe, I'm not providing guidelines, but garbanzo beans (chickpeas) and tahini (sesame seed paste) should be among the first three ingredients. Two tablespoons run around 45 calories, plus you're getting fiber, B vitamins, and other nutrients. Great as a sandwich filler or dip.

MILK AND SOY MILK

Train your palate to accept fat-free or 1% milk. If you're drinking 2% now, buy 2% and 1% and mix them for a few days or weeks, then gradually use less 2% and more 1% until you're comfortable with 1%. You can either stay there, or do the same mixing with fat-free (skim) until your taste buds adjust. Think fat-free milk is too watery? Don't worry; once you switch, you won't want to go back, as fattier milks will seem too heavy to you.

If you're lactose intolerant, you've got two good options: lactase-treated milk (such as Lactaid) and calcium-fortified soy milk. Again, go with the fat-free or 1% version of the lactase milk.

GUIDELINES FOR MILK OR SOY MILK
▶ **Serving size:** 1 cup
▶ **Calories:** No more than 110 calories
▶ **Calcium:** At least 25% of the DV

YOGURT

Low-fat plain yogurt is a wonderful food. It's richer in calcium than milk, easier to digest than milk for those with lactose intolerance, and the friendly bacteria cultures that turn milk into yogurt may offer some immune benefits. But sweetened, flavored yogurt is more of a dessert than a food, because of the heavy-handed use of sugar. Get this: 6 ounces (a typical single-serve carton) of plain, low-fat Dannon yogurt is 110 calories, with 13 g sugar (all naturally occurring milk sugar). That same size of a yogurt with fruit mixed in might have 150 calories and 26 g sugar; those extra 13 g sugar translate to 3¼ teaspoons added sugar! That's pretty much how it goes with all the brands, with some more sugary than others. All that sugar crowds out some of the calcium: 6 ounces plain yogurt supplies 300 mg (30% DV) while the sweetened yogurts offer 200 mg (20%).

If you like the sweetened, flavored yogurt, here's how to factor it into your *Supermarket Diet:* Count the first 100 calories as your daily calcium-rich serving, but all calories over 100 go toward your daily snack. So, 50 calories of a 150-calorie Dannon Fruit-on-the-Bottom yogurt comes out of your 125-calorie treat allowance on the Keep On Losin' plan, and 70 calories counts toward your treat if you have a 170-calorie Yoplait.

Or, eat the artificially sweetened (light) yogurts, which are about 100 calories per 6-ounce carton. They satisfy your daily calcium-rich serving without cutting into your treat calories. (Although you still get only 20% of the DV for calcium instead of 30% in plain yogurt.)

The most nutritious solution: Make your own fruit yogurt. You can control sugar, get more calcium, and have a little fresh fruit to boot. (For two quickie recipes, see pages 69 and 88.)

Deli Meat

Stick with the lean deli meats—turkey, chicken, lean ham, and roast beef—as opposed to bologna, salami, or "loaves," (such as ham-and-cheese loaf), which are high in saturated fat. If sliced at the deli counter, ask to see the label and compare to the guidelines below. Whenever possible, buy reduced-sodium products.

Fresh Fish

The fresher the fish, the less fishy the taste and the more delicious. Signs that fish is fresh: If you poke the flesh it should spring right back; it should not smell very fishy, and if you buy a whole fish, the eyes should be bright and not cloudy. Fattier fish provide healthy omega-3s but are higher in calories, so eat a smaller portion.

FISH WITH HIGHEST OMEGA-3 CONTENT (PER 4 OUNCES RAW)		
Fish	Calories/3 ounce serving	Omega-3s/3 ounce serving
Atlantic salmon, farm-raised	207	2.3 g
Atlantic salmon, wild	161	2.0 g
Trout, farm-raised	156	1.1 g
Trout, wild	135	0.8 g
Atlantic herring	179	1.9 g
Pacific herring	220	1.9 g
Bluefish	140	0.9 g
Bluefin tuna	163	1.3 g
Note: All types of salmon are high in omega-3s.		

Attention Shoppers! ➤ Fish Safety

You should eat fish, especially the fattier fish like salmon, sardines, and trout, because they're rich in omega-3 fats. These healthy fats help prevent heart disease and alleviate symptoms of depression and arthritis. Omega-3s are critical for the developing brain of the fetus; eating fish during pregnancy helps ensure that enough omega-3 is passed on to the developing infant.

However, there are contaminants in fish that limit the types and amount of fish pregnant women, women who might become pregnant, and young children can eat. For instance, certain types of fish are prone to high levels of mercury, which can cause neurological damage, especially in fetuses and children. Fish accumulate mercury by eating smaller fish, which have accumulated mercury by eating even smaller fish. So, the bigger the fish, the more mercury.

But you can eat fish safely, and you should. It's important that everyone, especially pregnant women, eat fish, so just follow the guidelines for the best and safest choices:

▶ Pregnant women and young children, breast-feeding women, women who might become pregnant: (1) Do not eat shark, swordfish, king mackerel, or tilefish (also referred to as golden bass or golden snapper) because they contain high levels of mercury. (2) Eat up to 12 ounces (two average meals) a week of a variety of fish and shellfish that are lower in mercury. Examples of low-mercury fish: anchovies, canned light tuna, catfish, cod, crab, freshwater trout, lobster, oysters, pollock, salmon, sardines, scallops, shrimp, and tilapia. (3) Canned albacore ("white") tuna has more mercury than canned light tuna. If you prefer albacore, then limit it to 6 ounces a week, as per the advice of the Food and Drug Administration. The FDA also recommends eating no more than 6 ounces of tuna steak weekly. In other words, have no more than 6 ounces weekly of either white albacore canned tuna or tuna steaks.

- The general population: Health authorities have not suggested that the rest of the population limit fish intake or even limit intake of the higher-mercury fish. To the contrary, the science shows that eating fish is good for you. The American Heart Association recommends eating *at least* two servings of fish per week. But to play it safe, limit your consumption of the higher-mercury fish listed above to once a month. Make sure to include other types of fish in your diet.
- Chemicals in farm-raised salmon: While the health authorities have not issued guidelines on farm-raised salmon for any member of the population—pregnant or not—research has found that it contains chemicals called organochloride compounds such as PCBs. These chemicals can harm the brain of the developing fetus, and long-term exposure to high levels of PCBs can increase cancer risk. Whether levels of PCBs in farm-raised salmon are high enough to hurt is still being debated. Wild salmon—the type in most canned salmon and the more expensive type found in the fresh fish section of the grocery store—is low in PCBs. For now, the best advice is go ahead and have farm-raised salmon, but make it just one of your fish meals each week. Enjoy other varieties of fish the rest of the week.
- For updated info, go the FDA's website at www.fda.gov and navigate your way to the fish advisories.
- Hate fish? Make sure to get plant-based omega-3s from products made with flaxseed (Nature's Path Flax Plus cereal and waffles are tasty examples). However, the plant form of omega-3, called alpha linolenic acid (ALA), isn't as potent a disease-fighter as the omega-3s in fish (called DHA and EPA). Some omega-3-enriched eggs have DHA, or a mix of DHA and ALA, so these would be helpful sources of the fat. If you have high blood triglycerides—a type of blood fat, like cholesterol, linked to heart disease—consult your doctor about whether you should take fish oil supplements.

Fresh Poultry

Any part of the chicken or turkey is fine, as long as you remove the skin. Or buy skinless. Buying ground turkey or chicken is tricky, because there isn't always a label, and if there is, you can't tell from the ingredient list whether skin is included. Grinding with the skin jacks calories and fat way up. If there's no label, ask at the poultry counter about ingredients.

COMPARE THE LABELS: GROUND TURKEY

Check out the differences in three kinds of raw ground turkey all from Shady Brook Farm, a brand found mainly on the East Coast. (Its sister company, Honeysuckle White, serves most of the rest of the country and has the same products.)

	Ground turkey, 15% fat (whole, includes skin)	Ground turkey, 7% fat (includes a little skin)	Ground turkey breast, 99% fat free (no skin, just breast meat)
Serving size	4 ounces (112 g)	4 ounces (112 g)	4 ounces (112 g)
Calories	220	160	120
Fat	15 g	8 g	0.5 g
Saturated fat	5 g	2.5 g	0 g

You can see that not all turkey is created equal. The inclusion of skin makes some turkey more fattening than others. Skip the high-fat ground turkey or chicken. If you're making chicken or turkey burgers, use the medium-fat variety (the guidelines following are for medium fat). The skinless ground breast will be too dry and crumbly for burgers but will work well mixed with beef in meatloaf, or by itself in bean chili or other mixed dishes.

Fresh Meat

The Supermarket Diet recipes specify the cuts of meat. You'll notice the recipes call for pork tenderloin, beef tenderloin (filet mignon), or beef top sirloin—the leaner cuts. Make sure to get them trimmed of visible fat, or do it yourself at home. The only time you'll need a fattier piece of meat is for making burgers. Leaner types of ground beef (95% or even 90% fat) make for a dry, crumbly burger. So use 85% fat ground beef for burgers, but make them an occasional treat because they're still high in saturated fat.

Precooked Poultry

The ultimate convenience food: no cooking, no defrosting. The catch: Much more sodium than if you made it yourself. When using these products, make sure you keep sodium low in the rest of the meal. Buy skinless chicken or turkey breast, and your numbers should look like this:

GUIDELINES FOR PRECOOKED SKINLESS CHICKEN AND TURKEY STRIPS (not breaded)
▶ **Serving size:** $1/2$ cup (71 g)
▶ **Calories:** 90 or less
▶ **Fat:** 2 g or less
▶ **Saturated fat:** 1 g or less
Compare these numbers to precooked, breaded chicken nuggets: For the same 71 g, you're stuck with around 180 calories, 11 g fat, and 3 g saturated fat.

Smoked Salmon

It tastes like a fatty and decadent treat, but it's actually a wonderfully nutritious food, rich in healthy omega-3 fats. Buy it in slices or as a shrink-wrapped little hunk of salmon (sometimes coated with peppercorns or another spice). No guidelines needed because it's all good stuff. The main difference between brands is whether they're preserved with nitrates/nitrites or not. These chemicals, if eaten regularly, may be linked to cancer.

Tortillas

I recommend whole-wheat tortillas throughout this book, but if you can't find them, buy the white-flour or corn type. While common in health food supermarkets, whole-wheat versions are still hard to find in mainstream grocery stores. Your guidelines: 120 to 130 calories per tortilla. You can use two 60-calorie tortillas if you don't find the 120-calorie type.

Part Three
Keeping It Off

8 Staying Slim: The Maintenance Program

You've lost weight. Congratulations! But now what? Well, that depends on your next goal: Do you want to keep losing, or do you want to maintain your weight loss? Read on to find out what to feed your body—and your mind—to meet either of these goals.

Knowing what to eat is important, but it's just half the weight-loss/maintenance battle. And by now—tutored by the Boot Camp and Keep On Losin' menus, plus all your new label-reading skills—you *do* know what to eat! You're *way* savvier about nutrition than most consumers. But what about your *attitude* toward losing weight?

There's a critical difference in attitude between people who maintain their weight loss and those who regain pounds. Many dieters who gain back all the weight they lost (and sometimes more) often view healthy eating and exercise as temporary activities to be endured just until the weight comes off. Then back to the bad old ways. People who maintain their weight loss see it differently, understanding that good eating habits are a lifelong activity and committing themselves to them. It might take a few tries before you arrive at the winning attitude, but stick with it for success.

In this chapter you'll find lots of ways to make "permanent" good eating habits appealing. Then use the Stay-Slim Maintenance plan as a healthy way of eating for life.

KEEP ON LOSIN' OR TAKE A BREAK?

Do you need to lose more weight? (Remember, be realistic. Squeezing into the jeans you wore senior year of high school is *not* a reasonable weight goal.) You can continue with the program, using the Keep On Losin' plan or take a break. Both approaches are legitimate. Let's say you started at 177 and you're down to 160, a fabulous 17-pound weight loss. That's about 10 percent of your body weight—gone! Some experts recommend holding steady at this weight for a while before losing any more. The reasons: to boost metabolism (which falls a little while you're losing weight) and to give yourself a psychological break from cutting calories. Often, a 10 percent loss of body weight is enough to improve cholesterol, blood sugar, and blood pressure. To maintain your current weight, you can probably move up to 1,700 or 1,800 calories. I'll show you how in this chapter. (But whatever you do, *keep exercising.*)

However, if you're still gung ho on the Keep On Losin' plan, stay on it. There's no rule that you must take a break. Read this chapter for tips to keep you motivated as you continue shedding pounds.

There is one danger to weight loss that you must avoid: becoming obsessed with thinness and continuing weight loss past a reasonable point. This obsession can turn into a serious eating disorder, such as anorexia or bulimia, both life threatening. How do you know when to stop losing? One clue is the BMI chart on page 260. Use the weight corresponding to a BMI of 19 as your stopping point. If you find yourself persistently dissatisfied with your body, obsessing about thinness, "feeling fat" despite being at a healthy weight (BMI under 25), then get professional help before you develop a full-fledged eating disorder, which can be difficult to shake.

EATING TO MAINTAIN

For women: You probably no longer need the 1,500-calorie Keep On Losin' plan if you're halting the weight loss. Whether you've reached your goal weight and want to maintain it or are just taking a break and maintaining an "in-between weight," you should be on about 1,700 or 1,800 daily calories. This should work if you keep exercising. If you find you're gaining weight, then reduce your daily intake by going back to the 1,500-calorie plan and add another 100 calories a day (there are plenty of lists in this book to show you how). Or, stick with the 1,800-calorie plan outlined here and increase your amount of exercise.

SuperTip ➤ Weight Maintenance Gets Easier

The longer you maintain your weight loss, the easier it is. In an ongoing University of Pittsburgh and University of Colorado joint study of more than 3,000 people that began in 1993 called the National Weight Control Registry, the average registrant lost approximately *60 pounds* and maintained that loss for roughly *5 years*. Six years into their maintenance they found they enjoyed exercising and eating low-fat meals even more than they did when they first lost the weight. But even more important, successful maintainers report that it all—eating healthily, exercising, and all the other habits that keep you trim—gets easier. Researchers speculate that the "costs" of weight maintenance are lowered, making the process easier, and with less effort required, it's more likely that people keep it up.

For men: remember, you should follow Keep On Losin' for only two weeks, then switch over to this chapter's 1,800-calorie plan to continue to lose weight. After you've lost the weight you've desired, you'll be able to convert this 1,800-calorie plan into a maintenance plan by adding 300 calories a day.

You get even more variety on the Stay Slim Maintenance plan than on Keep On Losin'. Now you can have any of the Keep On Losin' meals—just tack on more calories. Plus you've got even more higher calorie meals to choose from. The Keep On Losin' plan is chock full of vitamins, minerals, and other healthful compounds, and the meals are easy to prepare. That plan, like this one, is training you how to eat for the rest of your life. Remember: You're creating a plan you can live with for the long term. So, tailor it to your daily rhythm. If you want more variety and don't feel like supplementing the Keep On Losin' recipes, then consider the delicious Stay Slim recipes starting on page 226.

Here's a quick rundown of what you can expect on the Stay Slim Maintenance plan.

Breakfast: If the Keep On Losin' breakfasts have been working for you, stick with them. Or try adding 50–100 calories to those breakfasts (see list below). For some people, a bigger breakfast helps control calories and cravings the rest of the day.

Lunch: Lots of choices. Have any of your favorite Keep On Losin' lunches (all 400 calories), but bump up calories at breakfast and dinner. Or, add another 100 calories to any of those lunches. Or, have any of the 500-calorie Stay Slim Maintenance lunches in this chapter.

Dinner: Same drill as lunch. Either keep your favorite Keep On Losin' dinners (all 500 calories) and increase calories at breakfast and lunch. Or, add 50-100 calories to those dinners. Or, try the 550-600 calorie Stay Slim Maintenance dinners in this chapter.

Calcium Breaks: Leave 'em be, just as they are in the Keep On Losin' plan. Have one calcium treat a day. Keep taking your multivitamin with 200 to 300 mg calcium. If you're over age fifty, take a 200- to 500-mg calcium supplement as well.

Snacks: Ah, here's where it gets fun. See how many calories are left after you've fashioned a balanced plan. For example, if you upped breakfast to 475 calories, lunch to 500 calories, dinner to 550 calories, plus the 100-calorie calcium snack, your tally is 1,625. That leaves 175 calories for a snack. Cap the snack at 200 calories daily, though. You'll find a recommended list of snacks on page 216.

BIGGER BREAKFASTS

To move up from the 375-calorie breakfasts of the Keep On Losin' plan, simply add another 50 to 100 calories with these foods:

Bread, 1 slice (about 75 calories)
Cereal: add 50 or 100 calories

SuperTip ➤ Eat Your Breakfast!

About 90 percent of the successful dieters in the National Weight Control Registry eat breakfast regularly. This is in keeping with other studies showing that, all other things being equal, breakfast eaters are thinner than breakfast skippers. Some research indicates that cereal for breakfast—hot or cold—gives you an even greater weight-control edge.

While you might think that foregoing breakfast would keep calories lower all day, the practice backfires. Skip breakfast and your body gets wise eventually, demanding those calories later in the day, often in the evening or at a late hour when the last thing you feel like doing is preparing a salad or other healthful meal. So, you pig out on junk food, go to bed full, which makes you less hungry for breakfast in the A.M., and the vicious cycle continues.

Another plus from breakfast: a sharper mind. Studies of children and adults find memory and problem-solving skills are better after breakfast than when you skip the meal.

Egg, 1 (75 calories) If you have high cholesterol, check with your doctor about how many eggs you can eat per week. (Although most studies don't show a connection between egg consumption and blood cholesterol, some people may be more sensitive.)
Fruit: 1 large apple, pear, or banana (100 calories)
Margarine, trans fat–free, 1 teaspoon (40 to 50 calories)
Nuts, 1 heaping tablespoon (50 calories)

BIGGER LUNCHES AND DINNERS

Here are healthful ways to tack on extra calories to the 400-calorie Keep On Losin' lunches and 500-calorie Keep On Losin' dinners. You can add up to 100 calories to either meal or to both meals. Remember that you are increasing your total calorie intake by 200 to 300 calories, so if you've boosted your breakfast calorie consumption, then you are more limited about adding to lunch and dinner.

Men, when you're ready for a weight-maintenance plan, simply use this list to add calories to the lunch and dinner menus offered in this chapter. This will bring you up to about 2,100 calories, which should be ideal for maintenance. If it's still too low, double these additional portions. For instance, add ⅔ cup beans or ½ avocado to a meal.

Avocado, ¼ (85 calories)

Beans: Black beans, garbanzo beans, or other beans, a heaping ⅓ cup (100 calories)

Bread: Instead of 65- to 75-calorie bread, make sandwiches with bread that's about 90 calories per slice. Keep it whole grain!

Cheese, reduced-fat, 1 ounce (75 calories)

Chicken breast, no skin, ⅓ cup diced cooked (75 calories)

Corn, 1 medium ear (5 inches long) or heaping ½ cup whole kernels (80 calories)

Crackers: Check the label for calories and have a few more crackers with your soup.

Parmesan, grated, 1 tablespoon (23 calories): This small amount adds loads of flavor to salads, cooked vegetables, soups, and pasta.

Oil, olive, 1 teaspoon (40 calories)

Pasta, whole wheat, heaping ½ cup cooked (about 80 calories)

Peanut butter: Increase to 2 tablespoons from 4 teaspoons (65 calories, 1 tablespoon is 90 calories)

Rice, ⅓ cup cooked (about 80 calories)

Salad dressing, 1 tablespoon (typically 50 to 75 calories, check label to be sure)

80- TO 100-CALORIE MUNCHIES

Beverages

Beer, light

Milk, fat-free or 1% milk or soy milk, such as Silk or other brand (check labels), 1 cup

Wine, red, 4 ounces

Vegetable juice (V8), 12 ounces

Dairy

Cheese, reduced-fat Cheddar or Swiss, 1 ounce
Cheese, cottage, low-fat, 1/2 cup
Cheese, Gouda, Monterey Jack, Brie, 1 ounce
Yogurt, low-fat, 6 ounces

Fruit

Apricots, 5 dried
Banana, 1 small
Blueberries, fresh, 1 cup
Grapes, 25
Kiwi, 2
Pear or apple, 1 medium
Raisins, 3 tablespoons
Mango chunks, 1 cup
Watermelon chunks, 2 cups

High-Protein Foods

Burger, veggie, 1
Egg, 1
Chicken drumstick, without skin, 1
Peanut butter, 1 tablespoon
Peanuts or almonds, 15
Turkey breast, 3 oz.

Savory

Bagel chips, baked, New York–style (check label for calories), 5
Melba toasts, 4
Pretzels, Rold Gold Tiny Twist, 15
Soup, Amy's Butternut Squash or Cream of Tomato (both "Light in Sodium"), 1 cup
Soup, Health Valley Rich & Hearty Chicken Noodle, 1 cup
Tortilla chips, bite-size, Baked Tostitos, 18
Vegetable snack, dried, Just Veggies, 1 ounce (1/2 cup)

Starchy Comforts

Bread, cinnamon-raisin, 1 slice

Cereal, 50 calories worth (check label) with $1/2$ cup fat-free milk

Chili, vegetarian (check label for calories)

Rice or couscous, plain, cooked in broth, or mixed with fresh herbs, $1/2$ cup cooked

Waffle, frozen, Kashi GoLean, 1 (with 1 teaspoon maple syrup)

Sweets

Caramels, 3

Chocolate chips, 40

Chocolate-covered peanuts, 4

Fig Newtons, Nabisco, fat-free, 2

Frozen fruit bar, FrozFruit, 1

Fudgesicle, 1

Hershey's Kisses, 4

Jell-O Gelatin cup or fat-free pudding cup, 1

Raisinets (chocolate-covered raisins), 12

Rice Cakes, Quaker Caramel, 2 large or 7 mini

Vegetables

Asparagus or broccoli, 1 cup cooked, with 1 teaspoon olive oil

Avocado, $1/3$ cup

Baby carrots, 15

Cherry or grape tomatoes, 20

Fifteen Secrets of Successful Losers

With so many meals to choose from on the Stay Slim Maintenance plan, you'll never be at a loss for what to eat. And, hopefully, you've figured out an effective exercise strategy. Now the hard part: sticking with it. How can you turn around that temporary "I'm on a diet" mindset into lifelong healthful habits? Here are fifteen tried and true secrets from research studies of successful "losers" and from some of my own clients. This is your arsenal against gaining back the weight; use it!

SECRET #1: KEEP A FOOD DIARY

Uh oh, you've stopped losing, perhaps even started *gaining* weight! How come? Find out by putting pen to paper and jotting down everything you're eating. You can use the Food Diary on page 269. Either photocopy a few pages or simply write down the headings on a sheet of paper.

You may be in for a surprise. "Oops! Those little snacks—2 mini chocolate bars here, some handfuls of nuts there—are tacking on an extra 200 calories daily!" Or "Wow, I guess there has been too much wine this week." Or "Too much eating out." Your food diary will show you what you've been overdoing and also what you've been "underdoing." Skipped meals, not enough fruits and vegetables (which add satisfying bulk with few calories), meals that leave out an entire food group (like carbs) set you up for overindulging later.

SECRET #2: TELL YOURSELF, "FOOD IS NOT ENTERTAINMENT"

Sure, food can be entertaining, but always keep in mind that its primary role is to nourish you. When you stop using food as a form of entertainment—to rescue you from boredom, for instance—you'll start dropping pounds. Your food diary will clue you into when you're most vulnerable to using food for entertainment. When you find yourself eating for the wrong reasons, look elsewhere for a lift.

SECRET #3: USE FOOD-FREE METHODS TO SOOTHE AND COMFORT YOURSELF

In the same way you may use food to entertain yourself, you may also use it to help cope with sadness, excitement, anger, or numbness. Any emotion can be an eating trigger. But food is a dangerous source of relief, giving you temporary comfort while insidiously causing real grief in the form of excess weight. If you've been using food for years to cope with emotions, it's hard to change overnight. But take a stab at it: Eventually, your new approach will become second nature. Keep a list handy of nonfood activities that will remind you how to cope. Here are a few non-food–related activities that can help:

- Call a friend
- Take a walk
- Read a magazine, newspaper, or novel
- Browse the web
- Organize a drawer
- Do a crossword puzzle
- Write in your diary
- Watch a favorite TV show
- Go to the movies
- Listen to music
- Your suggestion here: _____

SECRET #4: SCHEDULE EXERCISE

Your calendar is essential for planning exercise. If you don't plan it into your week—*whoosh*—a zillion other events will pre-empt the time. Whether it's 20 minutes on your exercise bike at home, a 40-minute walk, or going to the gym, write it into your calendar. Exercise has *got* to be one of your priorities.

SECRET #5: HAVE EASY ACCESS TO EXERCISE

If your gym is a traffic jam away, or your creaky old exercise bike sits in a cluttered part of the basement, how much exercise are you really going to get? Cancel the membership at the gym in your old neighborhood, and join a gym closer to your home or office. Or move the bike upstairs (in front of the TV is a great spot). Making exercise easily accessible is critical.

SECRET #6: NIP WEIGHT GAIN IN THE BUD

Once a week, step on a scale, or try on a snug pair of jeans, or put a measuring tape to your waist. Use one of these measures to gauge body weight. The *minute* you find you've gained a few pounds, take action. (Re-measure a day later to make sure the gain was not simply a normal fluctuation in water weight.) Any pounds gained back are hard to lose.

SuperTip ➤ Move It!

National Weight Control Registry members exercise regularly, burning on average 2,827 calories per week. That's the equivalent of walking 28 miles a week! (Women's average was 2,800 calories expended a week through exercise; men 3,500 calories a week.) Using a stationary bike, walking, taking aerobic classes, jogging, and using stair-stepper machines were the favorite ways to keep trim.

Even people who have successfully maintained a big weight loss have a heck of a time shedding even two or three regained pounds.

SECRET #7: MINIMIZE HIGH-CALORIE BEVERAGES

Sugary sodas, alcohol, and even juices are a waste of calories. Have them if you love them, but they come straight out of the "snacks" allowance (125 calories on Keep On Losin' and 125 to 200 on the Stay Slim Maintenance plan). Here's the problem: Your body doesn't get full on liquid calories nearly as fast as it does on solids. So, it's easy to drink them *on top* of your regular intake. A 12-ounce can of soda, juice, or regular beer is about 150 calories; light beer is 100 calories per 12 ounces; and 4 ounces of wine is 83 calories. Remember, an additional 250 calories per day translates into a half pound a week in weight gain. About juice: It's always better to eat the whole fruit instead of juice, because you get fuller on fewer calories while chalking up fiber. If you'd like, it's OK to add a splash (2 to 3 tablespoons) of juice to seltzer.

SECRET #8: KEEP A WELL-STOCKED KITCHEN

Even if you're down to a few critical foods—some pasta, a jar of spaghetti sauce, a bag of frozen vegetables, and cold cuts—you can make yourself a nutritious meal in the 400- to 600-calorie range. That saves hundreds of calories over the fast-food meal you pick up because "there's nothing to eat at home." Keep your kitchen stocked with the foods recommended in "The Svelte Kitchen," chapter 2.

Super Tip ➤ Deal with Depression

It's hard to maintain your weight loss to the precise pound; even those in the National Weight Control Registry usually see about a five-pound "regain" over a two-year period. Some gained back even more, although they all stayed well below their initial weight. The main difference between those who could get rid of regained pounds and those who couldn't: depression. People who were depressed before regaining had a lot more trouble losing the pounds. The depressive symptoms were classic: feeling more tired or sad than usual, more aches and pains, difficulty focusing, and losing interest in things they once enjoyed. Besides all the other drags on your life, depression may upset your weight maintenance—another reason to acknowledge and address the blues before they sabotage all that you've accomplished.

SECRET #9: KEEP A POORLY STOCKED SUPPLY OF JUNK FOOD

Keep the boxes of cookies, pretzels, chips, and ice cream out of the house. Remember: Make junk food snacking an inconvenience. And if you *do* go out to get yourself that snack, bring home just one serving.

SECRET #10: WALK IT OFF

Sure, you could park in front of the store, shop, get back in your car, drive a half mile away, and park again in front of the bank. But don't. Leave the car in the parking lot equivalent of left field, walk to the store, shop, then *walk* to the bank and back to your car. That's calories burned, mood elevated, appetite suppressed, and chores done! Look for any other opportunities to burn calories: taking the stairs rather than the elevator, walking up escalators, walking instead of taking the subway (if you live in a city). Just an extra 100 calories burned each day (and you might end up burning lots more) translates to nearly a pound shed almost effortlessly each month.

SECRET #11: HANG OUT WITH LIKE-MINDED FRIENDS

Someone who'll meet you at the gym, or go on a walking date, or say no to dessert with you at a restaurant is an invaluable companion. Together, you can keep each other honest, encourage each other and make staying in shape enjoyable. Find online weight-loss buddies on the www.good housekeeping.com Weight Loss Support Group. Watch out for so-called friends who try to sabotage your weight loss by tempting you with scale-hiking foods!

SECRET #12: SEE A PROFESSIONAL

If you can afford a few sessions with a dietitian or a personal trainer, all the better. The dietitian can analyze your food records in a more precise way than you can, pointing out daily calorie intake, weak spots, and strengths. You can work with the dietitian on tweaking *The Supermarket Diet* meals to your own tastes while preserving calories and nutritional balance.

A personal trainer will show you how to safely use weights and give you an appropriate exercise regimen. If you've been a longtime couch potato and find it hard to get in the swing of exercise, making an appointment with a personal trainer may be just the jump start you need.

SECRET #13: "CHEAT" A LITTLE

Don't let that french fry or cookie craving build up to the point of a binge. Remember, you've got a 125-calorie daily snack allowance on the Keep On Losin' program and up to 200 calories on the Stay Slim Maintenance plan. Use that allowance to have reasonable portions of foods you love every day so you don't fall into the deprivation/binge cycle.

SECRET #14: HAVE LOW-CALORIE MUNCHIES ON HAND

When you need to nibble, think outside the junk food box. There are plenty of other foods that can make satisfying little snacks. There are foods to fit any craving, even healthy ones. Buy the smallest-size package possible of the more tempting snacks. And only keep *one* of those in the house.

SECRET #15: CONGRATULATE YOURSELF!

Whether you've lost 2 pounds or 200 pounds, take a minute each day to acknowledge your achievement. Whatever you do, don't berate yourself for not losing more weight. This could make you feel so bad that you'll go right out and drown your sorrows in candy bars. Remember, if you weren't losing—or even holding steady—odds are you'd be gaining weight. Think of creative ways to recognize your accomplishment. One of my clients put a brown grocery bag in her kitchen. For every pound she lost, she placed a 1-pound can of beans, soup, or other food in the bag. When she'd collected 10 pounds, she donated the bag to her community food bank. The impact of seeing—and lifting—those 10 pounds was awe-inspiring and made her proud.

Stay Slim Menus

500-CALORIE LUNCHES

In your 1,700- to 1,800-calorie Stay Slim Maintenance program, you can now introduce even more variety into your meals. You can elect to supplement the Keep On Losin' meals with an extra 100 calories in the ways suggested above or you can try the delicious lunches that follow. Like most of the other lunches in *The Supermarket Diet,* most of these take under 25 minutes to prepare. Some take a little longer for when you've got more time. As with the Keep On Losin' plan, fiber values are noted to help you create meal plans that add up to a total of 25 g fiber per day. All of the following meals are 500 calories. Recipes start on page 227.

Hot Meals

Black Bean–Vegetable Hash with tomato and fruit (14 g fiber)
Huevos Rancheros with salad (13 g fiber)
Skillet Beans and Rice (21 g fiber)
Vegetarian Tortilla Pie with vegetable or fruit (16 g fiber)

Salads

Chicken and Fruit Salad with bread (7 g fiber)
Horseradish Potato Salad with Roast Beef, with a smoothie (8 g fiber)
Niçoise Salad with bread (6 g fiber)
Sesame Chicken Salad, with soba noodles (5 g fiber)
Tex-Mex Cobb Salad with bread (14 g fiber)
Salmon and Bean Salad with pita and crudités (12 g fiber)

Sandwiches

BBQ Pork Sandwich and Light Slaw with applesauce (11 g fiber)
Bistro Chicken-Eggplant Sandwich with salad (8 g fiber)
Falafel Sandwich with tomato salad (12 g fiber)
Mediterranean Chicken Sandwich with salad and fruit (9 g fiber)

550- TO 600-CALORIE DINNERS

Since you're the designer of your 1,800-calorie maintenance plan, you can have or enhance a 500-calorie Keep On Losin' dinner or you can select one of the 550- or 600-calorie meals below. Like most of the other dinners in *The Supermarket Diet*, most of these take under 25 minutes to prepare, but some take a little longer (again, for when you have more time). As always, look at each meal's fiber count and try to make your daily fiber add up to 25 g or more. Since these dinners range from about 550 to 600 calories, exact calorie counts are noted on each. You'll find all the recipes starting on page 242.

Beef, Lamb, Pork, and Veal

Moroccan-Style Lamb with Couscous (13 g fiber, 598 calories)
Orange-Ginger Pork Medallions with mashed potatoes and escarole (9 g fiber, 544 calories)

Tuscan-style Steak and Beet, Orange, and Watercress Salad, with bulgur (14 g fiber, 555 calories)

Veal with Tomato and Arugula Salad, with bread (3 g fiber, 567 calories)

Chicken and Turkey

Rotisserie chicken with mashed potatoes and vegetables (8 g fiber, 553 calories)

Spicy Guacamole-Chicken Roll-Ups with fruit (20 g fiber, 579 calories)

Turkey Chili with corn bread and salad (13 g fiber, 586 calories)

Fish

Five-Spice Salmon with Asian Rice and salad (9 g fiber, 594 calories)

Pasta and Rice

Linguine with White Clam Sauce, with broccoli and fruit (10 g fiber, 559 calories)

Orzo with Shrimp and Feta, with Garlicky Spinach (7 g fiber, 564 calories)

Pasta with Tuna Puttanesca, with salad (11 g fiber, 593 calories)

Ravioli with salad (8 g fiber, 588 calories)

Rice Salad with Black Beans, with yogurt-topped fruit (17 g fiber, 549 calories)

Sesame Noodle and Chicken Salad, with fruit (15 g fiber, 589 calories)

Tofu Stir-fry with fruit (12 g fiber, 546 calories)

500-Calorie Stay Slim Lunch Recipes

Again, you'll find that some of the recipes, particularly main dishes for dinner, yield more than one portion. *The Supermarket Diet* assumes that you may be cooking for more than one person. Remember—for family members who are not on the diet, you can simply increase the size of their portions. If you find you have leftovers, simply freeze them for later use.

500-Calorie Lunches

Black Bean–Vegetable Hash with tomato and fruit (14 g fiber)
Have 1 serving hash with a sliced tomato or other vegetable and tangerine or other small fruit.

▌ **Black Bean-Vegetable Hash**
Prep: 15 minutes ■ Cook: 30 minutes ■ Makes 4 servings

1½ pounds all-purpose potatoes (about 4 medium), peeled and
    cut into ½-inch cubes
2 tablespoons vegetable oil
4 ounces Canadian bacon, cut into ½-inch pieces
1 large red pepper, cut into ½-inch pieces
1 can (15 to 19 ounces) black beans, rinsed and drained
4 large eggs
salt and coarsely ground black pepper (optional)

1. In 3-quart saucepan, heat potatoes and enough water to cover to boiling over high heat. Reduce heat to low; cover and simmer until potatoes are almost tender, about 4 minutes. Drain.

2. In nonstick 12-inch skillet, heat oil over medium-high heat. Add Canadian bacon, red pepper, and potatoes; cook, stirring occasionally, until vegetables are tender-crisp and browned, about 15 minutes. Stir in black beans; heat through. Divide hash among 4 warm plates.

3. Meanwhile, in 10-inch skillet, heat 1½ inches water to boiling over high heat. Reduce heat to medium-low. One at a time, break eggs into custard cup, then, holding cup close to water's surface, slip each egg into simmering water. Cook eggs until desired doneness, 3 to 5 minutes. With slotted spoon, carefully remove cooked eggs, one at a time, from water; drain egg (still held in spoon) on paper towels. Top each serving of vegetable hash with 1 egg. Sprinkle eggs with salt and pepper, if you like.
Each serving: About 409 calories ■ 22 g protein ■ 48 g carbohydrate ■ 11 g fiber ■ 14 g total fat (3 g saturated) ■ 227 mg cholesterol ■ 488 mg sodium.

Huevos Rancheros with salad (13 g fiber)

Have 1 serving Huevos Rancheros with a green salad: 2 cups mixed greens with 1 tablespoon Lemon Dressing (or 80 calories of your favorite dressing).

▶ Huevos Rancheros
Prep: 8 minutes ■ Cook: 7 minutes ■ Makes 4 servings

> 1 can (15 to 19 ounces) black beans, rinsed and drained
> 1¼ cups mild or medium-hot salsa (about 11 ounces)
> ¼ cup water
> 4 large eggs
> 3 ounces shredded Mexican cheese blend or shredded Cheddar
> ¾ cup chopped fresh cilantro or parsley leaves for garnish
> 4 warm flour tortillas (preferably whole-wheat)

1. In 10-inch skillet, mix black beans, salsa, and water. Heat to boiling over high heat, stirring frequently.

2. One at a time, break eggs into custard cup and slip into skillet on top of bean mixture. Reduce heat to medium-low; cover and simmer until whites are completely set and yolks begin to thicken, about 5 minutes, or until eggs are cooked to desired firmness.

3. To serve, sprinkle bean mixture and eggs with shredded cheese. Garnish with chopped cilantro. Serve with warm tortillas.

TIPS: Eggs will keep their shape better if they are very fresh and cold. Also, when you add eggs to the black bean mixture, hold the cup as close to the skillet as possible so they will spread less.

Each serving: About 389 calories ■ 24 g protein ■ 45 g carbohydrate ■ 11 g fiber ■ 12 g total fat (6 g saturated) 235 mg cholesterol ■ 852 mg sodium.

▶ Lemon Dressing
Prep: 5 minutes ■ Makes about ¾ cup

> ¼ cup fresh lemon juice
> ½ teaspoon salt
> ¼ teaspoon ground black pepper
> ½ cup olive oil

In medium bowl, with wire whisk or fork, mix lemon juice, salt, and pepper. In thin, steady stream, whisk in oil until blended.

Each tablespoon: About 81 calories ▪ 0 g protein ▪ 0 g carbohydrate ▪ 0 g fiber ▪ 9 g total fat (1 g saturated) ▪ 0 mg cholesterol ▪ 97 mg sodium.

▶ **Skillet Beans and Rice** (21 g fiber)
Prep: 15 minutes ▪ Cook: 30 minutes ▪ Makes 5 servings

    ¾ cup regular long-grain rice
    1 tablespoon canola oil
    1 medium green pepper, cut into ½-inch pieces
    1 medium red pepper, cut into ½-inch pieces
    1 medium onion, chopped
    1 can (15 to 19 ounces) black beans
    1 can (15 to 19 ounces) pink beans
    1 can (15 to 19 ounces) garbanzo beans
    1 can (14½ ounces) stewed tomatoes or other canned tomatoes,
        preferably reduced sodium
    ½ cup bottled barbecue sauce
    1 cup water

  1. Prepare rice as label directs.
  2. Meanwhile, in 12-inch skillet, heat oil over medium heat. Add green and red pepper and onion and cook until vegetables are tender-crisp.
  3. Rinse and drain black beans, pink beans, and garbanzo. Add beans, tomatoes, barbecue sauce and water to pepper mixture in skillet; heat to boiling over high heat. Reduce heat to low; cover and simmer 15 minutes.
  4. When rice is done, stir rice into bean mixture. Serve hot.

Each serving: About 513 calories ▪ 25 g protein ▪ 93 g carbohydrate ▪ 21 g fiber ▪ 5 g total fat (1 g saturated) ▪ 0 mg cholesterol ▪ 699 mg sodium (if using reduced-sodium tomatoes).

Vegetarian Tortilla Pie with vegetable or fruit (16 g fiber)
Serve one fourth of the pie with 1 cup raw vegetables, or finish with a kiwi or other small piece of fruit.

▶ Vegetarian Tortilla Pie
Prep: 10 minutes ▪ Bake: 10 minutes ▪ Makes 4 servings

    1 jar (12 ounces) medium salsa
    1 can (8 ounces) no-salt-added tomato sauce
    1 can (15 to 16 ounces) no-salt-added black beans, rinsed and
        drained
    1 can (14 to 15 ounces) no-salt-added whole-kernel corn,
        drained
    ½ cup packed fresh cilantro leaves, coarsely chopped
    4 tortillas, preferably whole-wheat (120 to 130 calories each)
    6 ounces reduced-fat Monterey Jack cheese, shredded (1½ cups)

1. Preheat oven to 500°F. Spray 15½ by 10½-inch jelly-roll pan with nonstick cooking spray.

2. In small bowl, mix salsa and tomato sauce. In medium bowl, mix black beans, corn, and cilantro.

3. Place 1 tortilla in prepared pan. Spread one-third of salsa mixture over tortilla. Top with one-third of bean mixture and one-third of cheese. Repeat layering two times, ending with last tortilla.

4. Bake pie until cheese has melted and filling is hot, 10 to 12 minutes.
Each serving: About 465 calories ▪ 27 g protein ▪ 70 g carbohydrate ▪ 14 g fiber ▪ 10 g total fat (6 g saturated) ▪ 27 mg cholesterol ▪ 916 mg sodium.

SALADS
Chicken and Fruit Salad with bread (7 g fiber)
Have 1 serving of the salad with 1 medium slice crusty whole-grain bread (equivalent to a 5-inch-long slice of French bread) spread with 1 teaspoon trans fat–free margarine.

▶ Chicken and Fruit Salad
Prep: 30 minutes ▪ Makes 4 servings

1 cooked roasting chicken or rotisserie chicken (about
    2¼ pounds), chilled
1 bunch (10 to 12 ounces) spinach, tough stems trimmed
1 medium pink or white grapefruit
2 medium Red Delicious apples or other apples
¾ pound seedless green grapes
⅓ cup bottled poppy-seed salad dressing

1. Remove and discard skin and bones from chicken; tear chicken into bite-size pieces. Set aside 3 cups chicken; reserve remainder for another use. Chop 1 cup loosely packed spinach leaves; set remaining leaves aside. Cut peel and white pith. Holding grapefruit over large bowl to catch juice with sharp knife, cut out sections from between membranes from grapefruit; core and cut unpeeled apples into ¾-inch chunks.

2. In large bowl, combine 3 cups chicken, chopped spinach, grapefruit, apples, and salad dressing; toss to coat.

3. To serve, arrange remaining spinach leaves on platter; spoon chicken salad over spinach leaves.

Each serving: About 400 calories ▪ 29 g protein ▪ 38 g carbohydrate ▪ 6 g fiber ▪ 16 g total fat (3 g saturated) ▪ 79 mg cholesterol ▪ 244 mg sodium (sodium varies depending on amount contained in poppyseed dressing).

Horseradish Potato Salad with Deli Roast Beef, with smoothie
(8 g fiber)

▶ Horseradish Potato Salad with Deli Roast Beef
Serve with Mango-Strawberry Smoothie (See page 126 in the Keep On Losin' recipes.)
Prep: 10 minutes ▪ Cook: About 20 minutes ▪ Serves 4

2 pounds small red potatoes, not peeled
1 small bunch chives
½ cup reduced-fat sour cream
2 tablespoons prepared white horseradish
½ teaspoon salt
⅛ teaspoon coarsely ground black pepper
1 medium shallot, minced (about 2 tablespoons)
1¼ pounds thinly sliced deli roast beef

1. In 3-quart saucepan, place potatoes and *enough water to cover;* heat to boiling over high heat. Reduce heat to low; cover and simmer until potatoes are tender, 10 to 12 minutes. Drain; cool slightly.

2. Meanwhile, reserve some chives for garnish; cut remaining chives into ¾-inch pieces. In large bowl, whisk cut chives with sour cream, horseradish, salt, pepper, and shallot.

3. When potatoes are cool enough to handle, cut each in half or into quarters if large. Add warm potatoes to sour-cream dressing in bowl; with rubber spatula, stir gently until potatoes are evenly coated. Let potato mixture stand 30 minutes at room temperature, stirring occasionally.

4. Serve potato salad warm or cover and refrigerate up to 1 day to serve cold. To serve, arrange roast beef and potato salad on large platter. Garnish with reserved chives.

Each serving: About 308 calories ▪ 24 g protein ▪ 40 g carbohydrate ▪ 6 g fiber ▪ 6 g total fat (3 g saturated) ▪ 61 mg cholesterol ▪ 1,000 mg sodium (sodium will be closer to 500 mg if roast beef is reduced-sodium).

Niçoise Salad with bread (6 g fiber)
Have 1 serving salad with 1 medium slice crusty whole-grain bread (equivalent to a 5-inch-long slice of French bread) spread with 1 teaspoon trans fat–free margarine.

▶ Niçoise Salad
Prep: 35 minutes ▪ Cook: 25 minutes ▪ Makes 4 servings

    1 tablespoon white wine vinegar
    1 tablespoon fresh lemon juice
    1 tablespoon minced shallot
    1 teaspoon Dijon mustard
    1 teaspoon anchovy paste
    ¼ teaspoon sugar
    ¼ teaspoon coarsely ground black pepper
    3 tablespoons extravirgin olive oil
    1 pound medium red potatoes, not peeled, cut into ¼-inch-
        thick slices

8 ounces French green beans (*haricots verts*) or regular green
    beans, trimmed
1 head Boston lettuce, leaves separated
12 cherry tomatoes, each cut in half
1 can (12 ounces) light tuna packed in water, drained and
    flaked
2 large hard-cooked eggs, peeled and each cut into quarters
½ cup Niçoise olives

1. Prepare dressing: In small bowl, with wire whisk, mix vinegar,
lemon juice, shallot, mustard, anchovy paste, sugar, and pepper until
blended. In thin, steady stream, whisk in oil until blended.

2. In 3-quart saucepan, combine potatoes and *enough water to cover;*
heat to boiling over high heat. Reduce heat; cover and simmer until tender, about 10 minutes. Drain.

3. Meanwhile, in 10-inch skillet, heat *1 inch water* to boiling over high
heat. Add green beans; heat to boiling. Reduce heat to low and cook
until tender-crisp, 6 to 8 minutes; drain. Rinse with cold running water;
drain.

4. To serve, pour half of dressing into medium bowl. Add lettuce
leaves and toss to coat. Line large platter with dressed lettuce leaves.
Arrange potatoes, green beans, cherry tomatoes, tuna, hard-cooked
eggs, and olives in separate piles on lettuce. Drizzle remaining dressing
over salad.

Each serving: About 388 calories ▪ 28 g protein ▪ 28 g carbohydrate ▪ 5 g
fiber ▪ 19 g total fat (3 g saturated) ▪ 130 mg cholesterol ▪ 802 mg
sodium.

Sesame Chicken Salad, with soba noodles (5 g fiber)
Serve one fourth of the salad on top of 1 cup soba noodles (Japanese
buckwheat noodles) or whole-wheat spaghetti tossed with ½ cup grated
carrots and 1 teaspoon Oriental sesame oil.

▌Sesame Chicken Salad
Prep: 30 minutes ▪ Broil: 8 minutes ▪ Makes 4 servings

4 skinless, boneless chicken breast halves (about 1 pound)
½ teaspoon salt
¼ teaspoon pepper
3 tablespoons Oriental sesame oil
3 tablespoons peanut butter
1½ tablespoons reduced-sodium soy sauce
2 tablespoons seasoned rice vinegar
1½ teaspoons sugar
1 teaspoon grated, peeled fresh ginger
¼ teaspoon hot pepper sauce
1 garlic clove, finely minced
¼ cup water
2 green onions
1 small red pepper
½ seedless cucumber
1 bunch watercress, tough stems trimmed

1. Preheat broiler. Rub chicken with salt, pepper, and 1 tablespoon sesame oil. Place chicken in broiling pan without rack. Place pan in broiler at closest position to heat source; broil chicken until chicken loses its pink color throughout, about 4 minutes on each side. Set aside until chicken is cool enough to handle.

2. Meanwhile, prepare dressing: In large bowl, with wire whisk, mix peanut butter, soy sauce, vinegar, sugar, ginger, hot pepper sauce, garlic, remaining 2 tablespoons sesame oil, and water until blended.

3. Cut green onions, red pepper, and unpeeled cucumber into 2½" by ¼" long matchstick strips.

4. With fork, pull chicken breasts into long, thin strips. Add chicken strips to bowl with dressing; toss until chicken is evenly coated.

5. To serve, line each plate with equal portions of watercress topped with equal portions of soba noodles and chicken salad. Arrange red pepper, cucumber, and green onions on top of salad.

Each serving: About 314 calories ▪ 31 g protein ▪ 9 g carbohydrate ▪ 2 g fiber ▪ 18 g total fat (3 g saturated) ▪ 66 mg cholesterol ▪ 666 mg sodium.

Tex-Mex Cobb Salad with bread (14 g fiber)

Have 1 serving of salad with 2 slices whole-wheat bread, each spread with 1 teaspoon trans fat–free margarine.

▶ Tex-Mex Cobb Salad

Prep: 30 minutes ▪ Makes 4 servings

¼ cup fresh lime juice
2 tablespoons chopped fresh cilantro leaves
4 teaspoons olive oil
1 teaspoon sugar
¼ teaspoon ground cumin
¼ teaspoon salt
¼ teaspoon coarsely ground black pepper
1 medium head romaine lettuce (1¼ pounds), trimmed and
    leaves cut into ½-inch-wide strips
1 pint cherry tomatoes, each cut into quarters
12 ounces cooked skinless turkey meat, cut into ½-inch pieces
    (2 cups)
1 can (15 to 19 ounces) black beans, rinsed and drained
2 small cucumbers (6 ounces each), peeled, seeded, and cut into
    ½-inch-thick slices

1. Prepare dressing: In small bowl, with wire whisk, mix lime juice, cilantro, oil, sugar, cumin, salt, and pepper until blended.

2. Place lettuce in large serving bowl. Arrange tomatoes, turkey, black beans, and cucumbers in rows over lettuce. Just before serving, add dressing and toss.

Each serving: About 308 calories ▪ 36 g protein ▪ 29 g carbohydrate ▪ 10 g fiber ▪ 6 g total fat (1 g saturated) ▪ 71 mg cholesterol ▪ 225 mg sodium.

Salmon and Bean Salad with pita and crudités (12 g fiber)

Have 1 serving salad with 1 (6-inch) whole-wheat pita. Serve with 1 cup cauliflower or other vegetables dipped in 2 tablespoons light ranch dressing (or 80 calories of any other dressing.

▶ Salmon and Bean Salad
Prep: 15 minutes ▪ Makes 4 servings

2 green onions, sliced
1 can (16 ounces) small white beans, rinsed and drained
1 can (7½ ounces) red salmon, drained and flaked
1 stalk celery, thinly sliced
Vinaigrette Dressing (below)
lettuce leaves
celery leaves, for garnish

1. In large bowl, combine green onions, beans, salmon, and celery; toss gently. Let stand about 40 minutes before serving.

2. To serve, stir Vinaigrette Dressing and pour over salmon mixture; toss gently to coat. Line platter with lettuce leaves; top with salmon mixture. Garnish with celery leaves.

3. Serve immediately, or chill up to 24 hours.

Each serving: About 261 calories ▪ 17 g protein ▪ 27 g carbohydrate ▪ 6 g fiber ▪ 10 g total fat (2 g saturated) ▪ 23 mg cholesterol ▪ 403 mg sodium.

▶ Vinaigrette Dressing
In small bowl, with fork, mix *2 tablespoons wine vinegar, 2 tablespoons olive oil, ¼ teaspoon sugar, ¼ teaspoon dry mustard, ¼ teaspoon salt,* and *⅛ teaspoon pepper* until blended. Makes about 4 tablespoons.

Each tablespoon: about 32 calories ▪ 0 g protein ▪ 0 g carbohydrate ▪ 0 g fiber ▪ 3 g total fat (0 g saturated) ▪ 0 mg cholesterol ▪ 145 mg sodium.

SANDWICHES
BBQ Pork Sandwich and Light Slaw with applesauce (11 g fiber)
Have 1 sandwich and 1 serving slaw with 1 cup unsweetened applesauce.

▶ BBQ Pork Sandwiches with Light Slaw
Prep: 10 minutes ▪ Boil: 15 minutes ▪ Makes 6 servings

3 tablespoons light molasses
3 tablespoons ketchup
1 tablespoon Worcestershire sauce
1 teaspoon minced, peeled fresh ginger
½ teaspoon grated lemon peel
1 garlic clove, crushed with garlic press
2 small, whole pork tenderloins (1½ pounds)
6 whole-grain hamburger rolls (about 170 calories each)

1. Preheat broiler. In medium bowl, combine molasses, ketchup, Worcestershire, ginger, lemon peel, and garlic. Add pork; turn to coat.

2. Place pork on rack in broiling pan. Spoon any remaining molasses mixture over pork. Place broiling pan 5 to 7 inches from heat source; broil pork, turning once, until pork is browned and meat thermometer inserted in thickest part of tenderloin reaches 155°F, 15 to 20 minutes. Internal temperature of meat will rise to 160°F on standing.

3. To serve, thinly slice pork. Serve on hamburger rolls with any juices from broiling pan.

Each sandwich: About 359 calories ▪ 31 g protein ▪ 43 g carbohydrate ▪ 5 g fiber ▪ 7 g total fat (2 g saturated) ▪ 72 mg cholesterol ▪ 493 mg sodium.

▌ Light Slaw
Prep: 10 minutes ▪ Makes 6 servings

1 bag (16 ounces) shredded cabbage mix for coleslaw
3 medium carrots, peeled and shredded
1 green onion, chopped
¼ cup seasoned rice vinegar
¼ teaspoon salt
¼ teaspoon coarsely ground black pepper

In large bowl, combine cabbage mix, carrots, onion, vinegar, salt, and pepper; toss to mix well. If not serving slaw right away, cover and refrigerate up to 6 hours. Toss well before serving.

Each serving: About 63 calories ▪ 2 g protein ▪ 15 g carbohydrate ▪ 4 g fiber ▪ 0 g total fat (0 g saturated) ▪ 0 mg cholesterol ▪ 417 mg sodium.

Bistro Chicken-Eggplant Sandwich with salad (8 g fiber)
Have 1 sandwich with a salad: 2 cups mixed greens tossed with 1 tablespoon Lemon Dressing (page 228) or 80 calories of any other dressing.

▶ Bistro Chicken and Eggplant Sandwiches
Prep: 20 minutes ▪ Cook: 10 minutes ▪ Makes 4 servings

1 small eggplant (12 ounces)
1 medium red onion
1 teaspoon dried basil leaves
2 tablespoons plus 1½ teaspoons balsamic vinegar
2 tablespoons olive oil
¼ teaspoon salt
¾ teaspoon coarsely ground black pepper
2 teaspoons all-purpose flour
1 teaspoon dried parsley flakes
4 skinless, boneless chicken breast halves (about 1¼ pounds)
1 large round loaf crusty whole-grain bread
3 tablespoons Dijon mustard

1. Preheat oven to 500°F. Spray 15½" by 10½" jelly-roll pan with nonstick cooking spray.
2. Cut eggplant lengthwise into ½-inch-thick slices. Cut red onion crosswise into ½-inch-thick slices. Arrange eggplant and onion slices in single layer in prepared pan.
3. In cup, mix basil with 2 tablespoons vinegar, 1 tablespoon oil, ⅛ teaspoon salt, and ½ teaspoon pepper. Brush half of vinegar mixture over vegetables. Roast vegetables, turning once and brushing with remaining vinegar mixture, until tender and beginning to brown, 10 to 12 minutes.
4. Meanwhile, on sheet of waxed paper, mix flour, parsley flakes, remaining ⅛ teaspoon salt, and remaining ¼ teaspoon pepper; use to coat chicken breasts. In 12-inch skillet, over medium-high heat, heat remaining 1 tablespoon oil until hot. Add chicken and cook, turning once, until

chicken loses its pink color throughout, about 7 minutes. Holding knife almost parallel to the work surface, cut each breast half into 3 slices.

5. To serve, from center of loaf of bread, cut four ¾-inch-thick slices (reserve remaining bread for another use). Top bread with eggplant slices, slightly overlapping, onion slices, separated into rings, and chicken.

6. In cup, mix Dijon mustard with remaining 1½ teaspoons vinegar; drizzle over chicken.

Each sandwich: About 387 calories ■ 39 g protein ■ 32 g carbohydrate ■ 6 g fiber ■ 11 g total fat (2 g saturated) ■ 82 mg cholesterol ■ 1037 mg sodium.

Falafel Sandwich with tomato salad (12 g fiber)
Have 1 sandwich with 1 sliced tomato topped with 2 tablespoons crumbled feta or other cheese of your choice.

▶ Falafel Sandwiches
Prep: 10 minutes ■ Cook: 16 minutes ■ Makes 4 sandwiches

    4 green onions, cut into 1-inch pieces
    2 garlic cloves, each cut in half
    ½ cup packed fresh Italian parsley leaves
    2 teaspoons dried mint
    1 can (15 to 19 ounces) garbanzo beans, rinsed and drained
    ½ cup plain dried bread crumbs
    1 teaspoon ground coriander
    1 teaspoon ground cumin
    1 teaspoon baking powder
    ½ teaspoon salt
    ¼ teaspoon ground red pepper (cayenne)
    ¼ teaspoon ground allspice
    olive oil nonstick cooking spray (or 1 teaspoon olive oil to
        grease pan)
    4 (6- to 7-inch) pitas
    1 cup Tahini Dressing (see below)
    accompaniments (choose one or more): sliced romaine lettuce,
        sliced tomatoes, sliced cucumber, sliced red onion, plain low-
        fat yogurt

1. In food processor with knife blade attached, finely chop green onions, garlic, parsley, and mint. Add garbanzo beans, bread crumbs, coriander, cumin, baking powder, salt, ground red pepper, and allspice and blend until a coarse puree forms.

2. Shape bean mixture, by scant ½ cups, into eight 3-inch round patties and place on sheet of waxed paper. Spray both sides of patties with olive oil spray.

3. Heat nonstick 10-inch skillet over medium-high heat until hot. Add half of patties and cook, turning once, until dark golden brown, about 8 minutes. Transfer patties to paper towels to drain. Repeat with remaining patties.

4. Cut off top third of each pita to form pocket. Place warm patties in pitas. Serve with ¼ cup tahini sauce each and choice of accompaniments.

Each serving (with ¼ cup dressing): About 418 calories ▪ 20 g protein ▪ 72 g carbohydrate ▪ 11 g fiber ▪ 6 g total fat (1 g saturated) ▪ 4 mg cholesterol ▪ 652 mg sodium.

▶ Tahini Dressing
Prep: 10 minutes ▪ Makes 4 servings

　　1 cup plain low-fat yogurt
　　4 teaspoons lemon juice
　　4 teaspoons tahini (ground sesame paste)
　　pinch ground cumin
　　pinch salt

In small bowl (or in blender), combine yogurt, lemon juice, tahini, cumin, and salt; whisk until blended.

Each serving: About 70 calories ▪ 4 g protein ▪ 6 g carbohydrate ▪ 0.5 g fiber ▪ 4 g total fat (0 g saturated) ▪ 4 mg cholesterol ▪ 88 mg sodium.

Mediterranean Chicken Salad Sandwich with salad and fruit
(9 g fiber)
Have 1 sandwich with a quick chopped salad: ½ cup diced cucumber; ½

cup diced red pepper or tomato mixed with 1 tablespoon fresh basil, mint, or dill; 2 teaspoons olive oil; and a dash of balsamic vinegar. Have a tangerine or other small fruit for dessert.

▶ Mediterranean Chicken Sandwiches
Prep: 25 minutes ■ Cook: 10 minutes ■ Makes 4 sandwiches

> 1 teaspoon fennel seeds
> ½ teaspoon dried thyme
> ½ teaspoon salt
> ¼ teaspoon coarsely ground black pepper
> 4 medium skinless, boneless chicken breast halves
>   (1¼ pounds)
> ¼ cup Kalamata olives, pitted and finely chopped
> 3 tablespoons reduced-fat mayonnaise
> 1 loaf (8 ounces) crusty whole-grain bread
> 2 small tomatoes, each cut into 4 slices

1. Preheat grill.

2. In mortar with pestle, crush fennel seeds with thyme, salt, and pepper. Rub both sides of chicken breasts with spice mixture; set aside.

3. In small bowl, mix olives and mayonnaise. Cut bread crosswise into 4 equal pieces, then cut each piece horizontally in half. Spread olive mixture evenly on cut sides of bread; set aside.

4. Place chicken on hot grill rack over medium heat and cook, turning once, until chicken loses its pink color throughout, 10 to 12 minutes. Transfer chicken to cutting board.

5. To assemble sandwiches, slice chicken breasts crosswise into ¼-inch-thick slices. On bottom halves of bread, layer sliced chicken and tomatoes. Replace top halves of bread.

Each sandwich: About 359 calories ▪ 39 g protein ▪ 31 g carbohydrate ▪ 5 g fiber ▪ 9 g total fat (2 g saturated) ▪ 85 mg cholesterol ▪ 940 mg sodium.

550- to 600-Calorie Stay Slim Dinners

BEEF, LAMB, PORK, AND VEAL

▶ **Moroccan-Style Lamb with Couscous** (13 g fiber, 598 calories)
Prep: 20 minutes ▪ Cook: 1 hour and 45 minutes ▪ Makes 8 main-dish servings

> 1½ pounds trimmed, boneless lamb shoulder, cut into 1¼-inch pieces
> 2 tablespoons olive oil
> 2 garlic cloves, finely chopped
> 1½ teaspoons ground cumin
> 1½ teaspoons ground coriander
> 1 large onion (12 ounces), cut into 8 wedges
> 1 can (14½ to 16½ ounces) stewed tomatoes
> 1 cinnamon stick (3 inches)
> 1¼ teaspoons salt
> ¼ teaspoon ground red pepper (cayenne)
> 1 cup water
> 2 pounds sweet potatoes (3 large), peeled and cut into 2-inch pieces
> 1½ cups couscous (Moroccan pasta), preferably whole wheat
> 1 can (15 to 19 ounces) garbanzo beans, rinsed and drained
> 1 cup dark seedless raisins
> ¼ cup chopped fresh cilantro

1. Pat lamb dry with paper towels. In nonreactive 5-quart Dutch oven, heat 1 tablespoon oil over medium-high heat until very hot. Add half of lamb and cook until browned, using slotted spoon to transfer meat to bowl as it is browned. Repeat with remaining 1 tablespoon oil and remaining lamb.

2. To drippings in Dutch oven, add garlic, cumin, and coriander; cook 30 seconds. Return lamb to Dutch oven. Stir in onion, tomatoes, cinnamon stick, salt, ground red pepper, and water; heat to boiling over high heat. Reduce heat; cover and simmer, stirring occasionally, 45 minutes. Stir in sweet potatoes; cover and simmer 30 minutes longer.

3. Meanwhile prepare couscous as label directs.

4. Add garbanzo beans and raisins to Dutch oven. Cover and cook, stirring once or twice, until lamb and vegetables are tender, about 5 minutes longer.

5. Just before serving, stir cilantro into stew and remove the cinnamon stick. Serve lamb stew on couscous.

Each serving: About 598 calories ▪ 32 g protein ▪ 89 g carbohydrate ▪ 13 g fiber ▪ 14 g total fat (4 g saturated) ▪ 69 mg cholesterol ▪ 742 mg sodium.

Orange-Ginger Pork Medallions with mashed potatoes and escarole (9 g fiber, 544 calories)

Have 1 serving each of the pork, Low-Fat Mashed Potatoes, and Escarole with Raisins and Pignoli.

▸ Orange-Ginger Pork Medallions
Prep: 10 minutes ▪ Cook: 15 minutes ▪ Makes 4 servings

> 1 pork tenderloin (1 pound), trimmed
> 2 medium oranges
> 3 teaspoons canola oil
> ¼ teaspoon salt
> 3 green onions, thinly sliced
> 1 tablespoon grated, peeled fresh ginger

1. Pat pork dry with paper towels. Cut tenderloin crosswise into ¾-inch-thick slices. With meat mallet or rolling pin, between two sheets of plastic wrap or waxed paper, pound each slice of pork to ½-inch thickness.

2. From 1 orange, grate peel and squeeze ½ cup juice. Cut remaining orange crosswise into ½-inch-thick slices; cut each slice in half. Set aside.

3. In heavy 12-inch skillet, heat 2 teaspoons oil over medium heat until hot. Add pork, sprinkle with salt, and cook until browned and cooked through, about 2½ minutes per side. Transfer pork to platter; keep warm.

4. In same pan, heat remaining 1 teaspoon oil. Add green onions, ginger, and grated orange peel; cook until green onions are lightly browned and tender, 2 to 3 minutes. Add orange slices and juice to skillet; cook 1 minute. Return pork medallions to skillet; heat through.

Each serving: About 202 calories ■ 25 g protein ■ 9 g carbohydrate ■ 2 g fiber ■ 7 g total fat (2 g saturated) ■ 74 mg cholesterol ■ 204 mg sodium.

▌ Low-Fat Mashed Potatoes
Prep: 15 minutes ■ Cook: 25 minutes ■ Makes 4 servings

2 pounds Yukon Gold potatoes, peeled and cut into 1-inch pieces
¾ cup low-fat milk (1%), warmed
2 tablespoons olive oil
¾ teaspoon salt
⅛ teaspoon ground black pepper

1. In 4-quart saucepan, combine potatoes and *enough water to cover;* heat to boiling over high heat. Reduce heat; cover and simmer until tender, about 15 minutes. Drain.

2. Return potatoes to saucepan. Mash potatoes with warm milk, oil, salt, and pepper until smooth and well blended.

Each serving: About 240 calories ■ 6 g protein ■ 39 g carbohydrate ■ 5 g fiber ■ 7 g total fat (1 g saturated) ■ 2 mg cholesterol ■ 204 mg sodium.

▌ Escarole with Raisins and Pignoli
Prep: 10 minutes ■ Cook: 20 minutes ■ Makes 4 servings

1 tablespoon olive oil
1 garlic clove, finely chopped

1 large head escarole (1 pound), coarsely chopped
¼ cup golden raisins
¼ teaspoon salt
2 tablespoons pine nuts (pignoli), toasted

In 5-quart Dutch oven, heat oil over medium heat. Stir in garlic and cook just until golden, about 30 seconds. Stir in escarole, raisins, and salt; cover and cook 5 minutes. Remove cover and cook until escarole is tender and liquid has evaporated, about 10 minutes longer. Stir in pine nuts and remove from heat.

Each serving: About 102 calories ▪ 3 g protein ▪ 12 g carbohydrate ▪ 3 g fiber ▪ 6 g total fat (1 g saturated) ▪ 0 mg cholesterol ▪ 172 mg sodium.

Tuscan-Style Steak and Beet, Orange, and Watercress Salad, with bulger (14 g fiber, 555 calories)

Have the steak and salad with 1 cup cooked bulgur or heaping ¾ cup cooked brown rice.

▶ Tuscan-Style Steak

Prep: 5 minutes plus standing ▪ Cook: 20 minutes ▪ Makes 4 servings

1 beef sirloin steak, 1½ inches thick (about 1¾ pounds),
    trimmed
2 teaspoons olive oil
½ teaspoon dried rosemary
¼ teaspoon dried thyme
¼ teaspoon coarsely ground black pepper
salt
1 lemon, cut into wedges

1. Pat steak dry with paper towels. In cup, mix oil, rosemary, thyme, and pepper. Use to rub over steak.

2. Heat 10-inch skillet over medium-high heat until hot. Add steak; reduce heat to medium and cook, turning once, 20 minutes for medium rare, or until desired doneness. Sprinkle steak generously with salt; transfer to warm large platter. Let stand 10 minutes; keep warm.

3. Cut steak into thin slices and serve with lemon wedges.

Each serving: About 244 calories ■ 29 g protein ■ 0 g carbohydrate ■ 0 g fiber ■ 13 g total fat (4 g saturated) ■ 88 mg cholesterol ■ 219 mg sodium (if ¼ teaspoon salt remained on entire steak).

▶ Beet, Orange, and Watercress Salad
Prep: 30 minutes ■ Cook: 30 minutes ■ Makes 4 servings

> 5 medium beets without tops (about 2 pounds)
> 2 large oranges
> 2 tablespoons olive oil
> 2 tablespoons red wine vinegar
> 1½ teaspoons Dijon mustard
> ½ teaspoon sugar
> heaping ¼ teaspoon salt
> ⅛ teaspoon coarsely ground black pepper
> 1½ or 2 bunches watercress (about 12 ounces), tough stems
>   removed
> ½ medium red onion, thinly sliced

1. In 4-quart saucepan, combine beets and *enough water to cover;* heat to boiling over high heat. Reduce heat; cover and simmer until tender, about 30 minutes.

2. Meanwhile, grate ½ teaspoon peel from 1 orange. Cut peel and white pith from all oranges. Holding oranges over large bowl to catch juice, cut between membranes to release segments. Place segments in small bowl; set aside. Add olive oil, vinegar, mustard, sugar, salt, pepper, and orange peel to juice. With wire whisk or fork, mix until blended.

3. Drain beets and cool with running cold water. Peel and cut each beet in half, then cut each half into ¼-inch-thick slices.

4. To dressing in bowl, add beets, orange segments, watercress, and red onion; toss to coat.

Each serving: About 153 calories ■ 4 g protein ■ 21 g carbohydrate ■ 5 g fiber ■ 7 g total fat (1 g saturated) ■ 0 mg cholesterol ■ 128 mg sodium.

Veal with Tomato and Arugula Salad, with bread (3 g fiber, 567 calories)
Have 1 serving veal with 1 medium slice crusty whole-grain bread (equivalent to one 5-inch-long slice of French bread) spread with 1 teaspoon trans fat–free margarine.

▶ Veal with Tomato and Arugula Salad
Prep: 20 minutes ▪ Cook: 5 minutes ▪ Makes 4 servings

  2 teaspoons fresh lemon juice
  6 tablespoons olive oil
  1 teaspoon salt
  ¾ teaspoon freshly ground black pepper
  1 large tomato (12 ounces), coarsely chopped
  1 cup loosely packed basil leaves
  ¼ cup coarsely chopped red onion
  1 pound veal cutlets
  2 large eggs
  ½ cup all-purpose flour
  1 cup plain dried bread crumbs
  1 bunch arugula (10 ounces), trimmed, or 2 bunches watercress

  1. In medium bowl, combine lemon juice, 2 tablespoons oil, ½ teaspoon salt, and ¼ teaspoon pepper. Stir in tomato, basil, and onion; set aside.
  2. With meat mallet or rolling pin, between two sheets of waxed paper or plastic wrap, pound cutlets to ⅛-inch thickness. In pie plate, beat eggs with remaining ½ teaspoon salt and remaining ½ teaspoon pepper.
  3. Place flour on waxed paper; place bread crumbs on separate waxed paper. Dip cutlets in flour, then in egg mixture, then in bread crumbs.
  4. In nonstick 12-inch skillet, heat 2 tablespoons oil over medium-high heat until very hot. Add half of cutlets; cook until browned, about 1 minute per side. Transfer to platter large enough to hold cutlets in single layer; keep warm. Repeat with remaining 2 tablespoons oil and remaining veal.

5. Add arugula to tomato mixture and toss to combine. To serve, spoon tomato and arugula salad on top of hot cutlets.

Each serving: About 476 calories ▪ 30 g protein ▪ 27 g carbohydrate ▪ 2 g fiber ▪ 27 g total fat (5 g saturated) ▪ 166 mg cholesterol ▪ 264 mg sodium.

CHICKEN AND TURKEY

Rotisserie chicken with mashed potatoes and vegetables (8 g fiber, 553 calories)

Have a leg or a breast of cooked chicken, skin removed. Serve with 1 serving of Mashed Potatoes with Horseradish Cream and 2 cups vegetables of your choice (e.g., thawed frozen broccoli, cauliflower, carrot mix) sautéed in 2 teaspoons olive oil and ½ teaspoon chopped garlic.

▶ Mashed Potatoes with Horseradish Cream

Prep: 25 minutes ▪ Bake: 20 minutes ▪ Makes about 5 servings

    2 pounds Yukon Gold potatoes (about 6 medium), peeled and
        cut into 1-inch chunks
    ½ container (4 ounces) reduced-fat sour cream
    1½ tablespoons snipped fresh chives
    ¼ cup reduced-fat (2%) milk, warmed
    ½ teaspoon salt
    2 tablespoons light mayonnaise
    1 tablespoon bottled white horseradish
    ⅛ teaspoon coarsely ground black pepper

1. Preheat oven to 450°F. In 6-quart saucepan, combine potatoes and *enough water to cover;* heat to boiling over high heat. Reduce heat; cover and simmer until potatoes are tender, about 15 minutes. Drain.

2. Meanwhile, reserve 2 tablespoons sour cream and half of the chives for topping.

3. Return potatoes to saucepan. With potato masher, mash potatoes with milk, salt, and remaining sour cream and chives. Spoon potato mixture into shallow 2½-quart casserole.

4. In small bowl, combine mayonnaise, horseradish, pepper, and reserved sour cream and reserved chives; stir until blended. Spread horseradish mixture over mashed potatoes. Bake potatoes until hot and bubbly and top is lightly browned, about 20 minutes.

Each serving (about 1 cup): About 188 calories ▪ 5 g protein ▪ 33 g carbohydrate ▪ 4 g fiber ▪ 4 g total fat (2 g saturated) ▪ 14 mg cholesterol ▪ 303 mg sodium.

Spicy Guacamole-Chicken Roll-Ups with fruit (20 g fiber, 579 calories)

Have 1 roll-up with a kiwi or other fruit for dessert.

◗ Spicy Guacamole-Chicken Roll-Ups

Prep: 30 minutes ▪ Cook: 12 minutes ▪ Makes 4 roll-ups

  1 tablespoon olive oil
  4 medium skinless, boneless chicken breast halves (about
     1 pound)
  ¼ teaspoon salt
  ½ teaspoon coarsely ground black pepper
  2 medium avocados (about 8 ounces each), peeled and cut into
     small chunks
  1 medium tomato, chopped
  ¼ cup loosely packed fresh cilantro leaves, coarsely chopped
  4 teaspoons fresh lime juice
  2 teaspoons finely chopped red onion
  1 teaspoon adobo sauce from canned chipotle chiles* or
     2 tablespoons green jalapeño sauce
  4 burrito-size (10-inch) tortillas, preferably whole-wheat (about
     200 calories each), warmed
  2 cups sliced iceberg lettuce

---

*Canned chipotle chiles in adobo (smoked jalapeño peppers in a vinegary marinade) are available in Hispanic markets and some large supermarkets.

1. In 10-inch skillet, preferably nonstick, heat oil over medium-high heat until hot. Add chicken and sprinkle with salt and ¼ teaspoon pepper. Cook chicken, turning once, until chicken loses its pink color throughout, about 12 minutes. Transfer chicken to plate; set aside 5 minutes, or until cool enough to handle.

2. Meanwhile, in medium bowl, with rubber spatula, gently stir avocados, tomato, cilantro, lime juice, red onion, adobo sauce, and remaining ¼ teaspoon pepper until blended.

3. With fork, pull chicken into thin shreds. Place tortillas on work surface; spread evenly with guacamole. Place chicken on each tortilla, then top with lettuce. Roll tortillas around filling.

Each roll-up: About 532 calories ▪ 37 g protein ▪ 57 g carbohydrate ▪ 17 g fiber ▪ 18 g total fat (4 g saturated) ▪ 66 mg cholesterol ▪ 614 mg sodium.

Turkey Chili with corn bread and salad (13 g fiber, 586 calories)
Have 1 serving of Turkey Chili or 350 calories of canned turkey and bean chili. Add a 3″ by 2″ piece of corn bread (about 125 calories) and a salad: 2 to 3 cups mixed greens, 80 calories of dressing of your choice or 1 tablespoon Lemon Dressing (page 228).

▶ Turkey Chili
Prep: 20 minutes ▪ Cook: 20 minutes ▪ Makes 4 servings

> 1 tablespoon olive oil
> 1 medium onion, chopped
> 3 garlic cloves, finely chopped
> 1½ teaspoons chili powder
> 1 teaspoon ground cumin
> 1 teaspoon ground coriander
> ¼ teaspoon salt
> ¼ teaspoon coarsely ground black pepper
> 1 can (15 to 16 ounces) Great Northern or small white beans, rinsed and drained
> 1 can (14½ ounces) reduced-sodium chicken broth or 1¾ cups homemade

1 package (10 ounces) frozen lima beans
1 can (4 to 4½ ounces) chopped mild green chiles
8 ounces bite-size pieces cooked turkey meat (2 cups)
1 cup loosely packed fresh cilantro leaves, chopped
2 tablespoons fresh lime juice
lime wedges (optional)

1. In 5-quart Dutch oven, heat oil over medium heat. Add onion and cook, stirring often, until tender, about 5 minutes. Add garlic and cook 30 seconds. Stir in chili powder, cumin, coriander, salt, and pepper; cook 1 minute longer.

2. Meanwhile, in small bowl, mash half of beans.

3. Add mashed beans and unmashed beans, broth, frozen lima beans, green chiles, and turkey to Dutch oven; heat to boiling over medium-high heat. Reduce heat; cover and simmer 5 minutes.

4. Remove Dutch oven from heat; stir in cilantro and lime juice. Serve with lime wedges, if you like.

Each serving: About 351 calories ▪ 33 g protein ▪ 38 g carbohydrate ▪ 10 g fiber ▪ 8 g total fat (2 g saturated) ▪ 53 mg cholesterol ▪ 631 mg sodium.

FISH

Five-Spice Salmon with Asian Rice and salad (9 g fiber, 594 calories)
Have 1 salmon fillet with 1 serving Asian Rice or ¾ cup plain brown rice. Serve with an orange/avocado salad: 2 cups greens, 1 sliced small orange, and ¼ sliced avocado, mixed with 2 teaspoons olive oil, ½ teaspoon lemon juice, and 1 tablespoon orange juice.

▌ Five-Spice Salmon
Prep: 5 minutes ▪ Broil: 6 minutes ▪ Makes 4 servings

2 teaspoons Chinese five-spice powder
1 teaspoon all-purpose flour
½ teaspoon salt
¼ teaspoon cracked black pepper
4 pieces salmon fillet (4 ounces each), with skin

1. Preheat broiler. Grease rack in broiling pan. In small bowl, mix five-spice powder, flour, salt, and cracked black pepper. Use to coat flesh side of salmon fillets.

2. Place salmon fillets, skin side down, on rack in broiling pan. Place pan in broiler at closest position to heat source. Broil salmon, without turning, until just opaque throughout, 6 to 7 minutes.

Each serving: About 199 calories ▪ 21 g protein ▪ 1 g carbohydrate ▪ 0 g fiber ▪ 12 g total fat (2 g saturated) ▪ 59 mg cholesterol ▪ 292 mg sodium.

❱ Asian Rice

Prep: 5 minutes ▪ Cook: 40 minutes (20 minutes for white rice) ▪ Makes 4 servings

> 1 cup rice, preferably brown
> 1 cup reduced-sodium chicken broth
> 1 cup water (¾ cup for white rice)
> 2 green onions, chopped
> 2 teaspoons reduced sodium soy sauce
> ¼ teaspoon Oriental sesame oil.

1. In medium saucepan, combine rice, broth, and water; heat to boiling over high heat. Reduce heat; cover and simmer, without stirring or lifting lid, until rice is tender and liquid has been absorbed, 40 minutes (18 to 20 minutes for white rice). Remove from heat and let stand 5 minutes.

2. Add green onions, soy sauce, and sesame oil to rice; toss with fork to combine.

Each serving: About 180 calories ▪ 4 g protein ▪ 37 g carbohydrate ▪ 2 g fiber ▪ 2 g total fat (0 g saturated) ▪ 0 mg cholesterol ▪ 128 mg sodium.

PASTA AND RICE

Linguine with White Clam Sauce, with broccoli and fruit (10 g fiber, 559 calories)

Have 1 serving pasta with 2 cups broccoli flowerets sautéed in 2 teaspoons olive oil (with 1 small clove garlic, if desired). For dessert, have 1 cup strawberries or any other fruit.

▶ Linguine with White Clam Sauce

Prep: 30 minutes ▪ Cook: 20 minutes ▪ Makes 6 servings

½ cup dry white wine
2 dozen littleneck clams, scrubbed*
1 package (16 ounces) linguine or spaghetti, preferably
    whole-wheat
¼ cup olive oil
1 large garlic clove, finely chopped
¼ teaspoon crushed red pepper
¼ cup chopped fresh parsley

1. With a stiff-bristled brush or other sturdy scrubber, clean clams well under cold running water to remove sand.

2. In nonreactive 5-quart Dutch oven, heat wine to boiling over high heat. Add clams; cover and cook until clams open, 5 to 10 minutes, transferring clams to bowl as they open. Discard any clams that have not opened; set aside to cool.

3. Strain clam broth through sieve lined with paper towels; set aside. When cool enough to handle, remove clams from shells and coarsely chop; discard shells.

4. Meanwhile, in large saucepot, cook the pasta as label directs; drain.

5. In same clean Dutch oven, heat oil over medium heat until hot. Add garlic and crushed red pepper and cook, stirring occasionally, just until garlic turns golden. Stir in parsley, clams, and clam broth; heat just to simmering. Add pasta to Dutch oven and toss to combine.

Each serving: About 396 calories ▪ 17 g protein ▪ 54 g carbohydrate ▪ 7 g fiber ▪ 12 g total fat (1 g saturated) ▪ 20 mg cholesterol ▪ 34 mg sodium.

Orzo with Shrimp and Feta, with Garlicky Spinach (7 g fiber, 564 calories)

Have 1 serving orzo with 1 serving Garlicky Spinach (page 108).

▶ Orzo with Shrimp and Feta

Prep: 10 minutes ▪ Cook: 20 minutes ▪ Makes 4 servings

1½ cups (10 ounces) orzo (rice-shaped pasta)
1 tablespoon butter or trans fat–free margarine
1 clove garlic, minced
1¼ pounds medium shrimp, shelled and deveined, with tail part
of shell left on, if you like
½ teaspoon salt
⅛ teaspoon coarsely ground black pepper
3 medium tomatoes, coarsely chopped
4 ounces feta cheese, crumbled (1 cup)
2 tablespoons fresh basil or dill, chopped, or 1½ teaspoons dried
oregano

1. Cook orzo as label directs.
2. Meanwhile, in nonstick 10-inch skillet, melt butter or margarine over medium-high heat. Add garlic and sauté for 30 seconds; then add shrimp, salt, and pepper; cook, stirring occasionally, until shrimp turn opaque throughout, 3 to 5 minutes. Add tomatoes and cook, stirring, 30 seconds. Remove skillet from heat.
3. Drain orzo. Add orzo, feta and herbs to shrimp mixture; toss to combine.
Each serving: About 504 calories ▪ 36 g protein ▪ 59 g carbohydrate ▪ 4 g fiber ▪ 13 g total fat (6 g saturated) ▪ 170 mg cholesterol ▪ 559 mg sodium.

Pasta with Tuna Puttanesca, with salad (11 g fiber, 593 calories)
Have 1 serving pasta with a salad: 2½ cups mixed greens tossed with 80 calories of dressing or 1 tablespoon of Lemon Dressing (page 228).

▶ Pasta with Tuna Puttanesca
Prep: 15 minutes ▪ Cook: 25 minutes ▪ Makes 4 servings

1 package (16 ounces) rotini or medium shells, preferably
whole-wheat
3 tablespoons capers, drained and chopped
3 tablespoons finely chopped shallots

2 tablespoons red wine vinegar

1 tablespoon olive oil

½ teaspoon freshly grated lemon peel

½ teaspoon salt

¼ teaspoon coarsely ground black pepper

2 cans (6 ounces) light tuna in olive oil

2 bunches watercress (4 to 6 ounces each), tough stems
   trimmed

½ cup loosely packed basil leaves, chopped

1. In large saucepot, cook pasta as label directs. Drain, reserving ½ cup pasta water.

2. Meanwhile, in large bowl, with fork, mix capers, shallots, vinegar, oil, lemon peel, salt, and pepper until well combined. Add undrained tuna and watercress; toss.

3. In pasta saucepot, toss pasta, basil, tuna mixture, and reserved pasta water.

Each serving: About 488 calories ▪ 29 g protein ▪ 62 g carbohydrate ▪ 8 g fiber ▪ 14 g total fat (2 g saturated) ▪ 38 mg cholesterol ▪ 824 mg sodium.

Ravioli with salad (8 g fiber, 588 calories)

Cook 400 calories of beef or chicken ravioli (i.e. 1½ cups of Buitoni Classic Beef or Chicken and Roasted Garlic Ravioli) according to package directions. Top with ⅓ cup meatless spaghetti sauce (store-bought or Marinara Sauce, page 118). Serve with a salad: 2 cups mixed greens or spinach, 1 cup chopped vegetables of your choice, and 4 teaspoons dressing.

Rice Salad with Black Beans, with yogurt-topped fruit (17 g fiber, 549 calories)

Have 1 serving salad. For dessert, serve 1 sliced orange topped with honey yogurt (¼ cup plain low-fat yogurt mixed with 2 teaspoons honey). If oranges aren't in season, pick another fruit.

▌ Rice Salad with Black Beans

Prep: 20 minutes ■ Cook: 10 minutes ■ Makes 4 servings

¾ cup regular long grain rice
2 large limes
2 cans (15 to 19 ounces) black beans, rinsed and drained
1 bunch watercress, tough stems trimmed
½ cup bottled salsa
1 cup corn kernels cut from cobs (about 2 medium ears)
¼ cup packed fresh cilantro leaves, chopped
1 tablespoon olive oil
½ teaspoon salt
¼ teaspoon coarsely ground black pepper

1. Prepare rice as label directs. Bring rice to room temperature. (You can refrigerate to speed this up.) Meanwhile, from limes, grate ½ teaspoon peel and squeeze 3 tablespoons juice.

2. In large bowl, mix rice, black beans, watercress, salsa, corn, cilantro, oil, lime peel and juice, salt, and pepper; toss well. Cover and refrigerate if not serving right away.

Each serving: About 406 calories ■ 19 g protein ■ 75 g carbohydrate ■ 14 g fiber ■ 4 g total fat (1 g saturated) ■ 0 mg cholesterol ■ 219 mg sodium.

Sesame Noodle and Chicken Salad, with fruit (15 g fiber, 589 calories)

Have 1 serving salad with 1 orange or other piece of fruit.

▌ Sesame Noodle and Chicken Salad

Prep: 25 minutes ■ Cook: 15 minutes ■ Makes 4 servings

12 ounces linguine or spaghetti (preferably whole wheat)
6 ounces snow peas, strings removed, each cut crosswise into thirds
¾ cup very hot water
¼ cup creamy peanut butter

3 tablespoons seasoned rice vinegar
3 tablespoons soy sauce
1 tablespoon brown sugar
1 tablespoon minced, peeled fresh ginger
1 tablespoon Asian sesame oil
¼ teaspoon ground red pepper (cayenne)
1 small garlic clove, crushed
2 medium carrots, peeled and shredded
½ small head red cabbage, thinly sliced (3 cups)
1½ cups thin strips boneless, skinless, roasted chicken

1. Prepare linguine as label directs. During last minute of cooking, add snow peas. Drain linguine and snow peas; rinse with cold running water to cool. Drain again; set aside.

2. Prepare peanut butter sauce: In large bowl, with wire whisk or fork, mix hot water, peanut butter, vinegar, soy sauce, brown sugar, ginger, sesame oil, ground red pepper, and garlic until blended.

3. Add linguine, snow peas, carrots, cabbage, and chicken to bowl; toss to combine. If not serving right away, cover and refrigerate. If noodles become too sticky upon standing, toss with a little *hot water* until dressing is of desired consistency.

Each serving: About 528 calories ▪ 21 g protein ▪ 79 g carbohydrate ▪ 12 g fiber ▪ 16 g total fat (2 g saturated) ▪ 9 mg cholesterol ▪ 738 mg sodium.

Tofu Stir-Fry with fruit (12 g fiber, 546 calories)

Serve one fourth of the stir-fry over 1 cup cooked brown rice. Enjoy 1 orange or other piece of fruit for dessert.

▶ Tofu Stir-Fry

Prep: 25 minutes ▪ Cook: 15 minutes ▪ Makes 4 servings

1 cup hot water
3 tablespoons reduced-sodium soy sauce
1 tablespoon brown sugar
1 tablespoon cornstarch
4 teaspoons canola oil
3 garlic cloves, crushed with garlic press
1 tablespoon grated, peeled fresh ginger
⅛ to ¼ teaspoon crushed red pepper
1 bag (12 ounces) broccoli flowerets, cut into uniform pieces if
    necessary
8 ounces shiitake mushrooms, stems removed and caps sliced
    (substitute regular mushrooms if shiitakes are unavailable)
1 medium red pepper, cut into 1-inch pieces
1 package (15 ounces) extra-firm tofu, patted dry and cut into
    1-inch cubes
3 green onions, thinly sliced
¼ cup salt-free cashews or peanuts, coarsely chopped

1. In small bowl, whisk water, soy sauce, brown sugar, and cornstarch
until blended; set aside.

2. In deep nonstick 12-inch skillet, heat oil over medium-high heat
until hot. Add garlic, ginger, and crushed red pepper and cook, stirring
constantly, 30 seconds. Add broccoli, mushrooms, and red pepper.
Cover and cook, stirring occasionally, 8 minutes.

3. Add tofu and green onions and cook uncovered, stirring occasionally, 2 minutes. Stir soy-sauce mixture and add to skillet; heat to boiling.
Boil, stirring, 1 minute.

4. Remove from heat. Top with cashews and serve.

Each serving: About 265 calories ▪ 18 g protein ▪ 20 g carbohydrate ▪ 5 g
fiber ▪ 16 g total fat (2 g saturated) ▪ 0 mg cholesterol ▪ 491 mg sodium.

Appendix 1

BODY MASS INDEX TABLE (See next page.)
(Reprinted courtesy of the National Heart, Lung and Blood Institute)

Body Mass Index Table

Normal: BMI 19–24 | **Overweight:** BMI 25–29 | **Obese:** BMI 30–39 | **Extreme Obesity:** BMI 40–54

Body Weight (pounds)

Height (inches) / BMI	19	20	21	22	23	24	25	26	27	28	29	30	31	32	33	34	35	36	37	38	39	40	41	42	43	44	45	46	47	48	49	50	51	52	53	54
58	91	96	100	105	110	115	119	124	129	134	138	143	148	153	158	162	167	172	177	181	186	191	196	201	205	210	215	220	224	229	234	239	244	248	253	258
59	94	99	104	109	114	119	124	128	133	138	143	148	153	158	163	168	173	178	183	188	193	198	203	208	212	217	222	227	232	237	242	247	252	257	262	267
60	97	102	107	112	118	123	128	133	138	143	148	153	158	163	168	174	179	184	189	194	199	204	209	215	220	225	230	235	240	245	250	255	261	266	271	276
61	100	106	111	116	122	127	132	137	143	148	153	158	164	169	174	180	185	190	195	201	206	211	217	222	227	232	238	243	248	254	259	264	269	275	280	285
62	104	109	115	120	126	131	136	142	147	153	158	164	169	175	180	186	191	196	202	207	213	218	224	229	235	240	246	251	256	262	267	273	278	284	289	295
63	107	113	118	124	130	135	141	146	152	158	163	169	175	180	186	191	197	203	208	214	220	225	231	237	242	248	254	259	265	270	278	282	287	293	299	304
64	110	116	122	128	134	140	145	151	157	163	169	174	180	186	192	197	204	209	215	221	227	232	238	244	250	256	262	267	273	279	285	291	296	302	308	314
65	114	120	126	132	138	144	150	156	162	168	174	180	186	192	198	204	210	216	222	228	234	240	246	252	258	264	270	276	282	288	294	300	306	312	318	324
66	118	124	130	136	142	148	155	161	167	173	179	186	192	198	204	210	216	223	229	235	241	247	253	260	266	272	278	284	291	297	303	309	315	322	328	334
67	121	127	134	140	146	153	159	166	172	178	185	191	198	204	211	217	223	230	236	242	249	255	261	268	274	280	287	293	299	306	312	319	325	331	338	344
68	125	131	138	144	151	158	164	171	177	184	190	197	203	210	216	223	230	236	243	249	256	262	269	276	282	289	295	302	308	315	322	328	335	341	348	354
69	128	135	142	149	155	162	169	176	182	189	196	203	209	216	223	230	236	243	250	257	263	270	277	284	291	297	304	311	318	324	331	338	345	351	358	365
70	132	139	146	153	160	167	174	181	188	195	202	209	216	222	229	236	243	250	257	264	271	278	285	292	299	306	313	320	327	334	341	348	355	362	369	376
71	136	143	150	157	165	172	179	186	193	200	208	215	222	229	236	243	250	257	265	272	279	286	293	301	308	315	322	329	338	343	351	358	365	372	379	386
72	140	147	154	162	169	177	184	191	199	206	213	221	228	235	242	250	258	265	272	279	287	294	302	309	316	324	331	338	346	353	361	368	375	383	390	397
73	144	151	159	166	174	182	189	197	204	212	219	227	235	242	250	257	265	272	280	288	295	302	310	318	325	333	340	348	355	363	371	378	386	393	401	408
74	148	155	163	171	179	186	194	202	210	218	225	233	241	249	256	264	272	280	287	295	303	311	319	326	334	342	350	358	365	373	381	389	396	404	412	420
75	152	160	168	176	184	192	200	208	216	224	232	240	248	256	264	272	279	287	295	303	311	319	327	335	343	351	359	367	375	383	391	399	407	415	423	431
76	156	164	172	180	189	197	205	213	221	230	238	246	254	263	271	279	287	295	304	312	320	328	336	344	353	361	369	377	385	394	402	410	418	426	435	443

Source: Adapted from *Clinical Guidelines on the Identification, Evaluation, and Treatment of Overweight and Obesity in Adults: The Evidence Report.*

Appendix 2

Tear-Out Sheet: Product Guidelines

Take these pages with you as you shop in the supermarket. (You will also find them on www.goodhousekeeping.com where you can print them at your convenience.) They list guidelines for calories, fiber, sodium, and other nutrients for a range of foods that are mainstays of *The Supermarket Diet*. So, when you're trying to choose a pasta sauce, just pull out these pages and check the "Pasta Sauce" guidelines, and find a jar of sauce that meets the criteria. Ditto for other foods on your shopping list.

Canned and Dry Foods
Bread and Crackers

BREAD
- Calories: 60 to 75 per slice
- Dietary fiber: at least 2 g per ounce (29 g). For many breads, an ounce is about 1 slice.
- Ingredient list: The first ingredient should be a whole grain, with the word *whole* in front of the words *wheat, rye,* or another grain. Oats don't have to be preceded by *whole*. Also acceptable: a white-flour product with bran and germ added back.

CRACKERS
- Serving size: 1 ounce (29 g)
- Calories: 115 to 130
- Dietary fiber: at least 3 g
- Saturated fat: 0.5 or less
- Ingredient list: The first ingredient should be a whole grain, with the word *whole* in front of the words *wheat, rye,* or another grain. Oats don't have to be preceded by *whole*. Also acceptable: a white-flour product with bran and germ added back.

Cereal and Breakfast Bars

COLD CEREAL

- Fiber: At least 4 g per 100 calories (translates to at least 6 g fiber per 150 calories)
- Saturated fat: No more than 1 g per 100 calories (1.5 g per 150 calories)
- Sugars: Preferable, but not a must: no more than 5 g per 100 calories, or no more than 8 g per 150 calories. It's OK for cereals like Raisin Bran, with dried fruit in the ingredient list, to have more sugar, about 7 g per 100 calories (11 g per 150 calories). That's because some of that sugar comes from the dried fruit, which is also supplying fiber and nutrients. But some fruit-filled cereals add too much sugar, so compare labels; the health food store versions are usually more moderate.
- Ingredient list: Preferable, but not a must: 100 percent whole grain. Some cereals break down the whole grain, then reassemble it.

HOT CEREAL

- Ingredient list: 100 percent whole grain or whole grain plus bran and/or wheat germ. Examples of whole grains in the ingredient list: barley, brown rice, oats, quinoa, whole rye, whole triticale, whole wheat. Exception: Oat bran. It's just the bran, not the whole-grain oat, but oat bran has been proven to help lower cholesterol.
- Sugars: Less than 5 g per 100 calories
- Fiber: At least 4 g per 150 calories

BREAKFAST BARS

- Fiber: At least 4 g per bar or 3 g per 100 calories
- Saturated fat: No more than 1 g per 100 calories
- Sugars: Preferably no more than 6 g per 100 calories (However, if fruit is a major ingredient, it's OK for sugar to be higher because it's naturally occurring fruit sugar.)
- Ingredient list: Preferably contains whole wheat, oats, or other whole grain

Canned Goods

CANNED CHILI, PER CUP
- Calories: 210 or less
- Saturated fat: 1 g or less
- Sodium: 800 mg or less

PASTA SAUCE (RED SAUCE, SPAGHETTI SAUCE), PER HALF CUP
TRY FOR AT LEAST THREE OUT OF FOUR:
- Calories: 90 calories or less
- Fat: 4 g or less
- Saturated fat: 2 g or less
- Sodium: 600 mg or less

SOUP AND BROTH
- Fiber: Choose mainly bean-based soups with around 5 g or more fiber per cup.
- Sodium: Aim for soups with under 600 mg of sodium per cup; the lower the better. Many Tabatchnik soups, found in the frozen section, are relatively low-sodium.
- Skip the cream soups; they usually offer little nutrition and often lots of fat. An exception: aseptically packaged "cream" soups based on soy milk sold in Health Food Stores (for example Imagine, Pacific, and Whole Foods' 365 brand).
- Broths should be under 400 mg sodium per cup.

Condiments/Dressings

SALAD DRESSING
- Calories: Regular dressing should be 100 to 150 calories per 2 tablespoons, the serving size usually listed on the label. Reduced-fat/reduced-calorie dressing should be under 100 calories per 2-tablespoon serving

- Fat: Choose dressings based on olive oil or canola oil
- Sodium: Compare labels, choose those lower in sodium.

SOY SAUCE (LIGHT), PER TABLESPOON
- Sodium: 560 mg

PEANUT AND OTHER NUT BUTTERS
- 150 mg sodium or less per tablespoon

Frozen Foods
Chicken and Turkey

CHICKEN AND TURKEY BURGERS (PATTIES)
- Serving size: 1 burger, 4 ounces (113 g)
- Calories: 160 to 170
- Fat: 8 g or less
- Saturated fat: 2.5 g or less
- Protein: 21 g or more

Fish

FISH BURGERS (FISH PATTIES)
(These guidelines are averages because numbers vary depending on the type of fish.)

- Serving size: 1 burger, 3.2 ounces (91 g)
- Calories: about 100
- Fat: about 3 g
- Saturated fat: 0 to 1 g
- Protein: about 17 g

FISH FILLETS, UNBREADED
These guidelines are averages because numbers vary depending on the type of fish.

- Serving size: 3.8 ounces (108 g)
- Calories: about 110
- Fat: about 3 g
- Saturated fat: about 0.5 g
- Protein: about 17 g

Meals and Other

FROZEN MEALS

- Calories: At least 300 calories, ideally 300 to 400 calories.

Look for at least two of the following:

- Saturated fat: No more than 5g
- Fiber: 5 g or more
- Sodium: 600 mg or less
- Protein: At least 14 g
- Carbs: Not much more than 45 g

PIZZA

- Calories: 450 to 470. That's a dinner portion on the Keep On Losin' plan. Add a salad with ½ teaspoon olive oil—for another 45 calories—for a meal total of about 500 calories. (If you want pizza for lunch on the Keep On Losin' plan, have about 350 calories' worth.) Read labels very carefully; sometimes 450 calories is an entire small pizza, sometimes a third of a pizza, or another amount. Do the math!
- Saturated fat: 7 g or less per 450 calories, which works out to be about 2 g saturated fat per 100 calories
- Sodium: Compare labels; the lower the better. Good luck!
- Toppings: vegetables, chicken, ham. Don't even pick up pizzas with pepperoni, sausage, ground beef, or double cheese! An exception: Reduced-calorie pizzas, such as some of the Lean Cuisine Café Classics Pizzas, which manage to include pepperoni and sausage and keep saturated fat and calories low.

VEGETABLE BURGERS

- Serving size: 1 burger, 2.5 ounces (70 g)
- Calories: preferably 110 to 120 (If you like one of the lower-calorie burgers, such as Boca Original Burger for 70 calories, then have 1½ burgers.)
- Protein: 12 g or more
- Sodium: Preferably under 400 mg, but if all the other elements are in place, it's OK to exceed this.
- Ingredient list: Soy should be the first or second ingredient.

WAFFLES

- Serving size: 2 waffles
- Calories: 190 or less
- Fiber: 4 g or more
- Sugars: Preferably under 5 g

Refrigerated Foods

Dairy

CHEESE, REDUCED-FAT/REDUCED-CALORIE

- Serving size: 1 ounce (29 g)
- Calories: No more than 75
- Fat: No more than 4 g
- Calcium: At least 20% of the DV

CREAM CHEESE, REDUCED-FAT

- Serving size: 2 tablespoons (30 g)
- Calories: 60 to 70
- Fat: 4 to 5 g
- Saturated fat: 3 g

MILK OR SOY MILK

- Serving size: 1 cup
- Calories: No more than 110
- Calcium: At least 25% of the DV

TRANS FAT–FREE MARGARINE

- Serving size: 1 tablespoon (14 g)
- Calories: 70 to 80
- Total fat: 8 to 9 g
- Saturated fat: 2.5 g or less
- Trans fat: 0 g
- Sodium: 95 g or less

Deli

DELI MEATS

- Serving size: 2 ounces (56 g)
- Calories: 45 to 80. One reason calories vary is because some companies inject water into their product, adding weight, not calories. So, while one brand may seem more expensive, it may not be if you're getting more real meat.
- Saturated fat: 1.5 g or less
- Sodium: Preferably under 500 mg sodium

CHICKEN AND TURKEY, PRECOOKED SKINLESS STRIPS (NOT BREADED)

- Serving size: ½ cup (71 g)
- Calories: 90 or less
- Fat: 2 g or less
- Saturated fat: 1 g or less

Fresh Meat

FRESH GROUND CHICKEN, RAW

- Serving size: 4 ounces (112 g)
- Calories: 170 or less
- Fat: 11 g or less
- Saturated fat: 3.5 g or less

FRESH GROUND TURKEY, RAW

- Serving size: 4 ounces (112 g)
- Calories: 160 or less
- Fat: 8 g or less
- Saturated fat: 2.5 g or less

Beef: Top sirloin, tenderloin, flank steak, London broil, tenderloin, roast beef, ground beef 90% fat-free (with the exception of the occasional burger using 85% fat-free)

Veal: Roast or lean chop

Lamb: Roast or lean chop

Pork: Pork tenderloin

Appendix 3
Food Diary

To get the most accurate picture of your diet, record your daily intake as accurately as possible. Here are five days worth of diary pages. You can copy the page for future diaries or download them from *Good Housekeeping*'s website at www.goodhousekeeping.com. Remember, recording your emotions will help to discover poor eating habits that are connected to certain moods or occasions.

You'll find a sample entry below.

Time/Place _____8 a.m., kitchen_____ Hunger Level _3__

Food/Amount ____1¹/₃ cups Kashi GoLean, 1 cup skim milk_____

_¹/₂ cup blueberries, 2 tablespoons walnuts_____

_____

Emotions/Situation _Tired but feel good about the healthy breakfast_____

_____

Food Diary

Date _____

Time/Place _____   Hunger Level* _____

Food/Amount _____

_____

_____

Emotions/Situation _____

Time/Place _____   Hunger Level* _____

Food/Amount _____

_____

_____

Emotions/Situation _____

Time/Place _____   Hunger Level* _____

Food/Amount _____

_____

_____

Emotions/Situation _____

Time/Place _____   Hunger Level* _____

Food/Amount _____

_____

_____

Emotions/Situation _____

_____

*Hunger levels: 1 = full; 2 = not hungry, not full; 3 = hungry; 4 = very hungry; 5 = desperately hungry

Food Diary

Date _____

Time/Place _____ Hunger Level* _____

Food/Amount _____

_____

_____

Emotions/Situation _____

_____

Time/Place _____ Hunger Level* _____

Food/Amount _____

_____

_____

Emotions/Situation _____

_____

Time/Place _____ Hunger Level* _____

Food/Amount _____

_____

_____

Emotions/Situation _____

_____

Time/Place _____ Hunger Level* _____

Food/Amount _____

_____

_____

Emotions/Situation _____

_____

*Hunger levels: 1 = full; 2 = not hungry, not full; 3 = hungry; 4 = very hungry; 5 = desperately hungry

Food Diary

Date _____

Time/Place _____   Hunger Level* _____

Food/Amount _____

_____

_____

Emotions/Situation _____

Time/Place _____   Hunger Level* _____

Food/Amount _____

_____

_____

Emotions/Situation _____

Time/Place _____   Hunger Level* _____

Food/Amount _____

_____

_____

Emotions/Situation _____

Time/Place _____   Hunger Level* _____

Food/Amount _____

_____

_____

Emotions/Situation _____

_____

*Hunger levels: 1 = full; 2 = not hungry, not full; 3 = hungry; 4 = very hungry; 5 = desperately hungry

Food Diary

Date _____

Time/Place _____ Hunger Level* _____

Food/Amount _____

_____

_____

Emotions/Situation _____

Time/Place _____ Hunger Level* _____

Food/Amount _____

_____

_____

Emotions/Situation _____

Time/Place _____ Hunger Level* _____

Food/Amount _____

_____

_____

Emotions/Situation _____

Time/Place _____ Hunger Level* _____

Food/Amount _____

_____

_____

Emotions/Situation _____

_____

*Hunger levels: 1 = full; 2 = not hungry, not full; 3 = hungry; 4 = very hungry; 5 = desperately hungry

Food Diary

Date _____

Time/Place _____ Hunger Level* _____

Food/Amount _____

_____

_____

Emotions/Situation _____

Time/Place _____ Hunger Level* _____

Food/Amount _____

_____

_____

Emotions/Situation _____

Time/Place _____ Hunger Level* _____

Food/Amount _____

_____

_____

Emotions/Situation _____

Time/Place _____ Hunger Level* _____

Food/Amount _____

_____

_____

Emotions/Situation _____

_____

*Hunger levels: 1 = full; 2 = not hungry, not full; 3 = hungry; 4 = very hungry; 5 = desperately hungry

Appendix 4
Physical Activity Readiness
Questionnaire

Regular physical activity is fun and healthy and being active is very safe for most people. If you are between the ages of fifteen and sixty-nine and are planning to become more physically active than you are now, the Physical Activity Readiness Questionnaire (PAR-Q) will tell you if you should check with your doctor before you start. If you are over sixty-nine, and you are not used to being very active, check with your doctor.

Common sense is your best guide when you answer these questions. Please read the questions carefully and answer each one honestly: check YES or NO.

1. Has your doctor ever said that you have a heart condition and that you should only do physical activity recommended by a doctor?

2. Do you feel pain in your chest when you do physical activity?

3. In the past month, have you had chest pain when you were not doing physical activity?

4. Do you lose your balance because of dizziness or do you ever lose consciousness?

5. Do you have a bone or joint problem (for example, back, knee or hip) that could be made worse by a change in your physical activity?

6. Is your doctor currently prescribing drugs (for example, water pills) for your blood pressure or heart condition?

7. Do you know of any other reason why you should not do physical activity?

Informed Use of the PAR-Q: The Canadian Society for Exercise Physiology, Health Canada, and their agents assume no liability for persons who undertake physical activity, and if in doubt after completing this questionnaire, consult your doctor prior to physical activity. Source: Physical Activity Readiness Questionnaire (PAR-Q) © 2002. Reprinted with permission from the Canadian Society for Exercise Physiology. http://www.csep.ca/forms.asp.

If you answered YES to ONE OR MORE questions:

Talk with your doctor by phone or in person BEFORE you start becoming much more physically active or BEFORE you have a fitness appraisal. Tell your doctor about the PAR-Q and to which questions you answered YES.

You may be able to do any activity you want as long as you start slowly and build up gradually. Or you may need to restrict your activities to those that are safe for you. Talk with your doctor about the kinds of activities you wish to participate in and follow his/her advice.

If you answered NO to ALL PAR-Q questions:
You can be reasonably sure you can:

- Start becoming much more physically active, beginning slowly and building up gradually. This is the safest and easiest way to go.
- Take part in a fitness appraisal, an excellent way to determine your basic fitness so that you can plan the best way for you to live actively. It is also highly recommended that you have your blood pressure evaluated. If your reading is over 144/94, talk with your doctor before you become much more physically active.

When to Delay Becoming More Active:

- If you are not feeling well because of a temporary illness such as a cold or a fever, wait until you feel better, or
- If you are a woman who is or may be pregnant, talk to your doctor before you start becoming more active.

PLEASE NOTE: If your health changes so that you then answer YES to any of the above questions, tell your fitness or health professional. Ask whether you should change your physical activity plan.

Appendix 5: Useful Conversions and Food Equivalents

3 teaspoons = 1 tablespoon

2 tablespoons = $^1/_8$ cup

4 tablespoons = $^1/_4$ cup

16 tablespoons = 1 cup = 8 ounces

2 cups = 1 pint = 16 ounces

2 pints (4 cups) = 1 quart = 32 ounces

4 quarts = 1 gallon

1 quart = 1 liter (approximately)

1,000 milligrams (mg) = 1 gram (g)

1,000 g = 1 kilogram (kg)

29 g = 1 ounce (oz.)

16 ounces = 1 pound

2.2 pounds = 1 kg

1 teaspoon sugar = 4 g

1 teaspoon fat = 5 g (includes oil, margarine, butter or any other fat)

1 teaspoon salt = 2,325 mg sodium

Index

Nut Butter and Toast, 67
nutrition guidelines, 188–190, 261
shopping for, 188–190
shopping lists, 39, 43
starch servings and, 132–133
Breakfast bars, 182–183, 262
Breakfasts. *See also specific recipes*
  50 to 100 calorie foods, 214–215
  375-calorie, 80, 84–88
  Boot Camp plan, 50–53, 54–55, 56, 60, 61, 63, 66, 67, 69, 70, 72
  designing your own, 133
  importance of eating, 215
  Keep On Losin' plan, 80, 84–88
  Stay Slim Maintenance plan, 214–215
Bulgur Wheat, 113–114
Burritos
  Bean, 60
  Egg, 61
  Vegetarian Black Bean, 98
Butter/margarine, 89, 198, 267

Cafeteria meal, 90
Calcium breaks, 82, 122–124, 214
Calories
  100-calorie foods, 47
  1,200-a day. *See* Boot Camp plan (1,200 calories a day)
  1,500-a day. *See* Keep On Losin' plan (1,500 calories a day)

1,800-a day. *See* Stay Slim Maintenance plan (1,800 calories a day)
  controlling, by making meals, 20
  on nutrition labels, 152, 153, 154
  reducing and burning, 16
Carbohydrates
  components of, 157
  good, 16–17, 157
  low-carb shortcomings, 16
  nutrition facts/labels, 152, 153, 157–158
  starchy comforts, 218
  sugar, 153, 157–158
Carrot-Bran Muffins, 85–86
Cauliflower, Roasted, 109
Cereal
  Apple Oatmeal with Brown Sugar, 66
  Banana Oatmeal with Brown Sugar, 70
  breakfast bars, 182–183, 262
  cold, 183
  fruit and, 86
  higher-protein, 184
  hot, 88, 184–186
  nutrition guidelines, 26, 183–186, 262
  pantry stand-bys, 26
  shopping for, 183–186
  shopping lists, 39, 44
Cheeses, 22, 198–199
Chicken
  500-calorie dinners, 81, 106–110
  550- to 600-calorie dinners, 226, 248–250
  burgers, 192, 264
  in cans or pouches, 28, 172

with couscous and spinach, 107
  fast-frozen, 22
  fresh, 205–206, 267
  good vs. bad fat and, 64–65
  nutrition guidelines, 192, 205–206, 207, 264, 267
  precooked, 207
  salads. *See* Salad(s)
  shopping for, 172, 192, 205–206, 207
  shopping lists, 41, 45
Chicken recipes
  Bistro Chicken and Eggplant Sandwiches, 238–239
  Chicken Wrap, 54
  Curried Butternut Squash Soup with Spinach, Couscous and Chicken, 72–73
  Mediterranean Chicken Sandwiches, 240–242
  rotisseries, 69, 109, 248
  Spicy Guacamole-Chicken Roll-Ups, 249–250
  Texas Chicken Burgers, 109–110
Chili, Baked Potato Stuffed with, 89–90
Chili, canned, 180, 263
Chili, Turkey, 250–251
Chips and dip, 128
Chocolate Milk, 123
Chocolate syrup, 43
Chokeberries, 87
Cholesterol. *See* Fat(s)
Cinnamon-Apple Butter Toast, 58
Cocoa, buying, 186–187
Coffee/tea, 187–188
Condiments. *See* Spreads/condiments